Fabulo
FOOD for KIDS

Fabulous FOOD for KIDS

ROSAMOND RICHARDSON

PIATKUS

First published in 1992 by
Judy Piatkus (Publishers) Ltd
5 Windmill Street
London W1P 1HF

A catalogue record for this book is available from the British Library

ISBN 0–7499–1182–4
ISBN 0–7499–1194–8 (Pbk)

Designed by Sue Ryall

Typeset by Phoenix Photosetting, Chatham, Kent
Printed and bound in Great Britain by
Biddles Ltd, Guildford & King's Lynn

Contents

Introduction

Are you flagging at the prospect of endless thrice-daily sessions in the kitchen, amid the hurly-burly of family life? Are you beginning to suspect it of being aversion therapy? Is your ideas department empty? Are you worried about whether your kids are eating a healthy and balanced diet? If so, this book is quite possibly for you.

The principle behind most of the recipes is that they are labour-saving, quick to make, and fun to do – with or without help from the kids. The food is targeted to please them as well as to nourish them on a healthy diet: nothing is more dispiriting to the hard-working cook than a child who rejects its plateful with a downturned mouth and 'I don't like this.'

○ MAKING IT FUN

A good deal of psychology is required in feeding kids, and certain ingredients have to be disguised. One way of making a dish attractive to them is to invent a title for it that incorporates their current heroes, whether cartoon or nursery rhyme characters, TV or football stars, or their favourite games and pastimes. It's a good idea to write any successful names alongside the recipes, so that you remember what to call the dish next time. It worked for me with my three – two of them were really difficult feeders, and I had a lot of practice! Always make an effort to arrange the food in a tempting way on the plate, too, and you'll go a long way in the art of persuasion.

○ BABIES AND CONVALESCENTS

Many of the dishes use leftovers, which provide welcome short cuts and make economical use of your resources. I recommend feeding babies on puréed portions of some of the meals in this book – it introduces them to interesting tastes at an early age and I found that mine really enjoyed being fed in this way instead of on processed baby foods. Pureé your chosen dish in the blender to a very fine consistency, adding pure bottled spring water to thin out as necessary. Suitable recipes are marked with the symbol [B].

Feeding convalescent children on mild, comforting food goes a long way to restoring health after illness, and many of the recipes are suitable for this purpose. Those that are particularly suitable are marked with the symbol [C].

○ INGREDIENTS

All the ingredients used in the recipes are easily available and store well, and so long as you check your 'sell-by' dates, and observe freezing instructions, you should not need to worry about storage, and you can shop in a planned and economical way. See the 'Ingredients' section on page 6 for further details.

○ A HEALTHY DIET

Choosing healthy ingredients is the bottom line of a good diet. For example, choose products with no added sugar where possible, such as muesli, or canned fruit in natural juice; choose lean mince and other meats; and select really fresh looking vegetables and fruit – not limp or soft produce which has lost its sparkle and probably most of its vitamins.

Although it is perfectly fine to use cream occasionally, or mixed half and half with yogurt, get into the habit of using skimmed or semi-skimmed milk, and low-fat yogurts and cheeses. I have included quite a lot of cheese in the recipes, because kids generally love it and it is a good source of protein and calcium. So go for the low-fat cheeses whenever appropriate.

Always READ THE LABEL. You will very soon identify the offending 'E' numbers and additives. Avoid them. Give your children pure food: it is a good start in life.

There is no dispute amongst nutritionists and doctors that many allergies are caused by food products and especially additives. Hyperactivity is a classic syndrome of the additive freak: these things affect the brain. So go for wholesome, well-balanced meals for the kids, and feed them as little 'junk food' as possible. I have included home-made versions of pizzas, burgers, milk shakes and ice cream, so you have no excuse!

There is no great mystique about a healthy diet. The guidelines are: choose low fat produce, reduce your sugar intake, and avoid additives and processed foods. Buy fresh fruit and vegetables, and as much 'whole', unprocessed food as possible. Be aware of what you are giving your children in their food. But beware of becoming too obsessive: if you labour the health angle with your kids they are more likely than not to revolt and become secret burger-eaters and coke-drinkers.

○ VEGETARIANS

Many children today are choosing to be vegetarian. Allow them, they have a right to their choices. If you are worried by the protein question, rest assured that vegetarians can easily obtain more than the required daily intake of protein through dairy products, pulses and soya products. Baked beans on wholemeal toast is a splendid example of a perfectly balanced protein meal. Use silken tofu to blend sauces – it is packed with protein and is now available at major supermarket chains. Give them Marmite on their wholemeal toast so that they get the required vitamin B12, and check that they get enough fresh fruit and vegetables. Where recipes are given for meat and meat products, use vegetarian substitutes – there are tasty sausagemeat and mince or burger mixes, completely vegetarian, which work very well (see page 8).

○ FAMILY MEALS

Children appreciate good food just as much as adults: so why always make the distinction between cooking for children and then again for the adult section of the family? Many of the recipes in this book have proved as successful with the grown-ups as with the children, while at the other end of the spectrum there is baby enjoying them too.

One of the problems of having to cook every day without respite is dreaming up ideas of what to have: often we churn out the same old things. So I have divided the book up into different mealtimes to help you find new ideas easily, but there are no rules about what you should serve when. Many of the lunch dishes, for example, are just as successful served as supper dishes.

○ QUANTITIES

Equally well there are no rules for quantities: appetites vary enormously from child to child, and even from day to day. Thus not all of the recipes state the quantity they serve: this is a matter of personal consumption, but on average they are targeted to four helpings. The cook in charge will be the best judge of how much her clients will eat.

Bon appetit! Hopefully you will now find it possible to make your daily cooking inspired, and to provide wholesome, balanced and healthy food for all the family.

☆ *H*andy *H*ints ☆

○ EQUIPMENT

Indispensable in your armoury of kitchen gadgetry is a **set of scales**. Some swear by digital scales, but personally I recommend a set of wall scales which give both metric and imperial. Whenever you want to use them, they are ready: just pull down the weighing tray and the conversion table is there in front of your eyes. The tray is removable and washable, and when not in use the gadget is out of the way and unobtrusive on the wall.

I also find a **microwave oven** indispensable. I use it to defrost food from the freezer, and I use it to cook all my vegetables which it does inimitably. It is practical, quick, clean and easy to use – and it saves on the washing up because no saucepans are involved.

It is wonderfully useful for heating up leftovers. After reheating anything, allow the food to cool for at least as long as you heated it for. Before offering it to the kids make sure it's cool enough for their delicate palates.

Equally indispensable in my view is a **good food-processor**. I recommend one that has a small bowl as well as a large one, for chopping herbs and nuts and making breadcrumbs. Buy as many of the blades and slicers as you can afford – it is a wonderful investment. Coleslaw for ten takes 30 seconds, and that is what it's about. . . . These processors make inimitable soups, and do just about anything you ask of them.

You may possess a **mixer** or **hand-held electric beater**, and the latter I find particularly useful – it takes much of the time and sweat out of baking. I am convinced that this piece of equipment is the key to light cakes.

Other artillery

- A really good set of knives, with a handy knife-sharpener. They make ALL the difference to working in the kitchen.
- A rubber scraper to clean out bowls and saucepans.
- A food-thermometer – essential for deep-frying and handy for jams.
- A good can-opener – wall-mounted if you have a convenient spot in the kitchen.
- One of my favourites – a tomato knife – a long, thin, delicate serrated knife which cuts like a cheese cutter.

○ COLLECTING RECIPES

Early on in my cooking career I discovered an excellent way of collecting recipes and keeping them in usable order: keep them written out on cards in a box file which you divide into different categories – e.g. soups, pies, fish, salads, etc. This book has been developed from the collection I made in this way from my mother's recipes, friends' ideas, cuttings from magazines and so on. The card system is easy to use and can be neatly stored in a corner of the kitchen.

○ INGREDIENTS

Bacon

Buy lean bacon where possible, and heat it in a heavy pan without added oil, or only a very little, until its own fat has run and it starts to crisp.

When you are wrapping bacon around something, first stretch it with the back of a knife along a wooden board, until it is half the thickness and twice the length.

Breadcrumbs

I use breadcrumbs a lot in cooking, both as a topping and as an ingredient. I keep my leftovers and crusts in a plastic bag in the fridge, and when I have enough I blend them in the processor and dry them on a baking sheet in a slow oven.

As an alternative to using breadcrumbs as a topping you can use crumbled cheese crackers with a sprinkling of wheatgerm, or crushed potato crisps.

Cheese

Cheddar makes very good cooking cheese and is usually popular with the whole family. However, to ring the changes you can substitute Jarlsberg, Cheshire or Double Gloucester. Mozzarella is comparatively low in fats, but has to be sliced rather than grated and goes stringy when cooked. Parmesan is the best of the hard cheeses, and is ideal for use in toppings or for sprinkling over the finished dish.

There are also many excellent low- or reduced-fat cheeses on the market which are helpful in reducing your family's total fat intake. Some of them are made with skimmed milk. Read the label! For serious vegetarians, there are several cheeses made without animal rennet, and again it is necessary to read the information on the packaging.

Eggs

Use free range eggs, size 1 or 2.

When using a recipe that includes separated eggs, first beat the whites and then the yolks – in that order. This way there is no need to wash the beater in between.

If the recipe calls for only the whites or only the yolks, there is no need to waste the rest. Use whites for Banana Frost and Fire, or Polar Bear Pud, Banana and Orange Meringue or Infallible Meringues. Yolks come in handy for making quiches and flans, Mayonnaise and Truffles, and for enriching sauces. Both will store, covered, in the fridge for 24 hours.

Herbs

As the loving tender of a herb garden I am lucky enough to have access to fresh herbs for much of the year and I use them a lot in cooking. You don't have to grow herbs – many fresh herbs are available in our shops nowadays, and dried herbs are very effective. If using dried, you will need only half the quantity given for fresh herbs.

Which herbs you use is a question of personal taste – there are no hard and fast rules about which ones go best with which ingredients. Everyone has their preferences, and it is fun to keep experimenting.

Margarine

One of the ways to cut down on saturated fats in your kids' diet is to use polyunsaturated margarines. Sunflower is my preference – it has more flavour than soya, for example, and has a softer texture. But this is a matter of taste. Occasionally there are recipes where butter is called for, or where it makes a good alternative, and there is no harm in that. As with any 'healthy' diet, balance is the key.

Milk
I prefer to use semi-skimmed milk for everything. I prefer it as it's not too heavy and creamy on the one hand, nor too watery on the other. It also provides all the vitamins and calcium of whole milk with half the fat.

Nuts
I have not always specified which kind of nuts to use, since this depends on what I have in the larder as well as on my mood. The basic range covers walnuts, almonds, hazelnuts and dry-roasted peanuts. Choose according to taste and what is to hand.

Oil
Again this is a question of taste and mood. I like cooking with sunflower oil much of the time, because of its light, unobtrusive flavour. But when the fancy takes me I switch to olive oil. I also make all my salad dressings and mayonnaise with it.

For deep-frying, ground nut oil is definitely the best. It's tasteless, clean and light. Soya oil is also a good alternative to sunflower and ground nut oil.

Stock
You can make your own chicken, fish or meat stock in the traditional way, by boiling the bones with herbs and an onion in lots of water for up to an hour. Keep the pan covered.

If you are using stock cubes, use vegetable ones preferably; and read the label. The meat ones are sometimes made from unmentionable trimmings.

Sugar
Unless otherwise specified use unbleached granulated sugar.

Vegetarian substitutes
These have got better and better over the years, and are now

tasty and satisfying, and very easy to use. Follow the rehydration instructions on the packet, and then use in the recipes as if you were using the meat ingredient itself. If you feel that it needs more flavour, add some dried or fresh herbs to the mixture, and season well with sea salt and freshly ground black pepper.

Wholemeal or plain?

Faced with the choice of wholemeal or plain pasta, brown or white (polished) rice, wholemeal or plain flour, most kids will opt for the processed version. Undoubtedly wholemeal pasta and flour make for heavier dishes, and many children won't touch brown rice, which seems to be an acquired taste. My advice is to mix in small amounts of the wholemeal variety, giving the dish a healthy balance which is also acceptable to your child's palate. Yet again we are in the area of preference: some kids take to wholemeal more easily than others. You are the best judge.

○ REHEATING LEFTOVERS

If you are reheating leftovers in a steamer, or in the microwave, make sure that the food gets really hot. Never reheat anything twice.

○ GREASING CAKE TINS

Use oil to grease a cake tin or loaf tin. Smear it around so that the entire inner surface is lightly covered, then dust with flour. To do this, sprinkle a small amount of flour into the tin and knock it around from underneath so that the surface is completely covered, then knock out the residue. The baked cake will come out without a struggle.

Brilliant Breakfasts and Brunches

The first meal of the day often tastes the most delicious, and certain well-tried breakfast favourites never fail: hot buttered toast and jam (see pages 137–42 for delicious home-made jams and spreads); boiled egg and soldiers; home-made muesli with yogurt or milk; warm croissants, brioches or Danish pastries for an occasional treat; or the great British porridge. When it comes to brunch, and you have worked up even more of an appetite, food can taste incomparably good. In addition, brunch makes a refreshing break from the usual morning routine (i.e. nobody gets ticked off for getting up late). For the ravenous at mid-morning, these recipes will not fail to make mouths water.

Bubbling Grapefruit

This hot-and-cold variation of grapefruit makes a refreshing start to the day. A marmalade topping is bubbled under the grill, hardly heating the fruit segments below.

Per person
½ grapefruit
1–2 tbs marmalade of your choice

Loosen the grapefruit segments with a serrated knife and spread the tops with good home-made marmalade (see pages 137–8). Put under a hot grill for a minute or so until the marmalade bubbles. Serve immediately.

Golden Muesli

A crunchy, crisp version of muesli, with browned sunflower seeds and nuts, this is scrumptious with thick yogurt or milk.

Makes 2 lb (900 g)

12 oz (350 g) porridge oats
2 oz (50 g) bran
3 oz (75 g) barley kernels
2 tbs sunflower seeds
3 tbs chopped mixed nuts
¼ pint (150 ml) sunflower oil
¼ pint (150 ml) golden syrup
3 tbs currants

Preheat the oven to 180°C/350°F/gas mark 4. Mix together all the ingredients except the currants. Put the mixture into a large, shallow baking tray and bake for about 20 minutes, turning from time to time until lightly browned. Remove from the oven and stir in the currants. Allow to cool, then store in airtight jars.

Yummy Yogurts

There are some truly wonderful yogurts on the market nowadays: thick and creamy Greek yogurt; organic cow's-milk yogurt, live, with its slippery texture and unbeatable taste; and my favourite – thick sheep's-milk yogurt with its smooth texture and distinctive flavour.

Yogurt is very versatile. There are many ways of inventing your own special flavourings and mixtures to make a refreshing start to the day.

Try adding 2 large tbs muesli (see above) to 5 fl oz (150 ml) plain yogurt, and mix together in a bowl. Lovely just as it is, or with some grated apple. [C]

To flavour and sweeten plain yogurt, add 2 tbs clear honey, or jam – plum, blackcurrant, apricot and strawberry are particularly good. Mix together well and it is ready to eat. [B]

Fresh fruit mixed into yogurt is also delicious. Sliced bananas, chopped pears, fresh blackberries, sliced oranges or mandarin sections, or halved seedless grapes are all excellent. [C]

My favourite combination is sliced grapefruit segments: a refreshing start to the day which never fails to wake me up. As a variation, add some barley kernels as well – they add texture and body to the mixture.

ROLY POLY BACON

Chunks of banana are wrapped in thin bacon and baked so that the bacon is crisp. Served on fried bread, they make a memorable breakfast or brunch.

Per person
2 streaky bacon rashers, rinded
½ banana
1 slice wholemeal bread, fried in oil

Preheat the oven to 200°C/400°F/gas mark 6. Place the rashers flat on a board and 'stretch' them by pulling the back of a knife along their length. Cut the bananas into 2.5 cm (1 inch) chunks and wrap them in lengths of the stretched bacon rashers. Secure them with a toothpick, then bake for 15–20 minutes until the bacon is crisp. Serve on fried bread.

You can improvise with other fillings too: little rolls of sausage meat, leftover stuffing, or nuggets of fresh, lightly cooked fish.

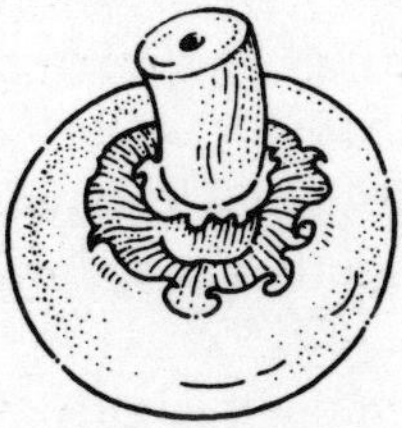

BACON AND MUSHROOM TOASTS

Mushroom-lovers, this one is for you! A piping-hot layer of mushrooms on toast is topped with crisp bacon.

Per person
1 slice wholemeal bread
sunflower margarine
2 rashers bacon
1½ oz (40 g) button mushrooms, chopped

Preheat the oven to 230°C/450°F/gas mark 8. Cut the crusts off the bread and spread one side of each slice with sunflower margarine. Grill, margarine side up, until a pale golden-brown. Spread the other side with more margarine and press browned-side down into a square ovenproof dish.

Fry the bacon until crisp, then cook the chopped mushrooms in the bacon fat until they are soft, adding a little margarine if necessary. Place the mushrooms on the toast, cover with the bacon and bake for 5 minutes. Serve piping hot.

EGGS WITH A HAT

A picturesque version of fried eggs on toast. The eggs are cooked inside a cut-out circle of fried bread, and topped with the missing round. Lovely served with grilled tomatoes.

Per person
1 slice granary bread
sunflower oil
1 egg
sea salt and pepper

Cut a round out of each slice of bread with a pastry cutter or small glass. Set the slices aside and fry the circles in oil until golden-brown on both sides. Place on a baking tray in a low oven to keep warm.

Begin to fry the remainder of the slices, and when golden-brown on one side turn them over. Break an egg into each hole and season it with salt and pepper. Continue cooking until the bread is golden on the underside and the egg lightly set.

Serve on warm plates with the cut-out rounds on top of the eggs.

Scrimble Scramble Ⓒ

This delectable mixture of bacon and scrambled eggs topped with cheese and onion makes a substantial breakfast or brunch dish.

Serves 2–4

4 rashers bacon
4 free-range eggs
a little sunflower oil
4 slices Cheddar cheese
4 thin slices onion
4 rounds wholemeal toast

Fry the bacon until it is crisp. Break the eggs into the fat, adding a little oil if necessary, and spread the bacon around the pan, breaking up the eggs with a fork. Put the slices of cheese on top and the slices of raw onion on top of that. When the cheese has melted, cut the mixture into four and serve on buttered toast.

SUNRISE SURPRISE

This is one of my family's favourite brunches. If you are cooking for vegetarians, use vegetarian sausage mix instead of the black pudding. Follow the packet instructions for reconstituting the mix first. It makes a real treat of those late, lazy weekend mornings.

Per person
3 oz (75 g) black pudding or sausage
1 egg, separated
a little milk
salt and pepper
1 tsp chopped fresh herbs
sunflower oil

Skin and grill the black pudding or sausage, until crisp on both sides. Drain on kitchen paper, cool, and crumble.

Beat the egg white until stiff. Beat the yolk with a little milk and season lightly. Add the crumbled black pudding or sausage and the chopped fresh herbs to the egg yolk, then fold in the stiffly-beaten white. Fry the mixture in sunflower oil in a heavy pan, over a moderate heat, until the bottom is golden, being careful not to let the outer edges burn. Cut into wedges and eat with fresh bread or croissants.

FARM FRY

A fry of bacon, potatoes and onions is bound together with lightly scrambled eggs for a satisfying brunch.

4 slices bacon, chopped finely
4 potatoes, peeled, boiled and cut into small dice
1 tbs chopped onion
salt and pepper
4 eggs

Fry the bacon until crisp. Drain off most of the fat, then add the potatoes, chopped onion, salt and pepper. Sauté until the potatoes are golden and softened. Break the eggs into the pan and stir until the eggs are set. Serve immediately on hot plates.

CRISPY CRACKLING FISH BITES

These deep-fried fish-balls are a real treat: they melt in the mouth and can be guaranteed to vanish as quickly as they are produced. The best thing about them is that they can be prepared the day before and cooked in no time at all next morning.

Makes 12

1 small onion, grated
1 oz (25 g) butter
1 oz (25 g) flour
¼ pint (150 ml) skimmed milk
12 oz (350 g) cod or haddock, cooked, boned and flaked
1 oz (25 g) fresh granary breadcrumbs
2 oz (50 g) Cheddar cheese, grated (optional)
a little beaten egg
salt and pepper
vegetable oil

Gently fry the grated onion in the butter for 5 minutes. Add the flour, stirring for 2 minutes, then gradually stir in the milk. Bring to the boil, stirring all the time, then lower the heat and simmer for 3 minutes. Add the fish, breadcrumbs, optional cheese, enough beaten egg to bring the mixture to a holding consistency, and salt and pepper. Stir thoroughly, allow to cool, and then chill.

Divide into 12 balls and deep-fry in hot oil (195°C/390°F) for 3–4 minutes until puffed and golden. Drain on kitchen paper and serve at once.

Irresistible Soups

Beautiful soup, so rich and green,
Waiting in a hot tureen!
Who for such dainties would not stoop?
Soup of the evening, beautiful soup!
Soup of the evening, beautiful soup!
Beau—ootiful Soo——oop!
Beau—ootiful Soo——oop!
Soo——oop of the e——e——evening,
Beautiful, beautiful soup.

From *Alice's Adventures in Wonderland*
by Lewis Carroll

There is nothing quite like soup for comforting, nourishing food – at all times and for all ages. Even when children go through tiresome stages of eating (or not eating), soup doesn't seem to raise the usual grumbles. Many of the soups here are labour-saving and can make quick and substantial meals in their own right, served with one of the breads on pages 25–6, or with some of the sandwiches on pages 107–9.

Creamy Broccoli Soup Ⓒ

A simple vegetable soup enriched with yogurt or cream. Delicious with the Emergency Loaf on page 25.

Makes 1½ pints (900 ml)

1 lb (450 g) broccoli florets
1 pint (600 ml) vegetable stock
4–5 tbs thick yogurt or cream
salt and pepper

Cook the broccoli florets until tender – I tend to use the microwave since it retains the flavour and colour of the broccoli so well. Cool. Put into the blender with the stock and whizz to a purée. Pour into a pan and heat gently. Finally stir in the yogurt or cream, season to taste, and serve without bringing it to the boil.

Onion Super-Soup

This is a wonderfully warming soup for cold weather, with golden grilled slices of French bread and cheese floating in it. A meal in itself.

Makes 1½ pints (900 ml)

2 oz (50 g) sunflower margarine
1 lb (450 g) onions, chopped
1 pint (600 ml) stock
salt, pepper and nutmeg
1 French loaf, sliced
3–4 oz (75–100 g) Cheddar cheese, grated

Melt the sunflower margarine in a saucepan, add the onions and toss them until well coated. Cover the pan with a lid, turn the heat right down and cook until soft and sweet, stirring occasionally. This will take 25–30 minutes.

Add the stock and bring to a simmer, stirring, then cook gently for 10 minutes. Season to taste. Pour into individual bowls, float the slices of bread on top and cover each one with grated cheese. Finish under a hot grill, until the cheese bubbles and turns golden.

CORN CAULDRON ©

Thick and golden, this nourishing soup is for all seasons. An excellent standby served with warm granary rolls.

Makes 1½ pints (900 ml)

12 oz (350 g) canned or frozen sweetcorn, thawed and drained
½ pint (300 ml) hot vegetable stock
½ pint (300 ml) milk
1 small onion, sliced
1 oz (25 g) sunflower margarine
1 tbs wholemeal flour
salt and pepper

Combine the corn, stock, milk and onion in a saucepan and simmer over a low heat for 10–15 minutes. In another pan melt the sunflower margarine. Stir in the flour and gradually add the hot corn mixture. Bring to the boil and simmer for a few minutes. Liquidise and season to taste. Thin out with more milk if necessary, reheat and serve.

WATERCRESS COTTAGE POTTAGE ©

This fresh country soup made with watercress is one of the most popular with my children. They love it with the Bread Fingers on page 25.

Makes 2 pints (1.2 litres)

2 bunches watercress
2 oz (50 g) sunflower margarine
1½ pints (900 ml) stock
salt
2 oz (50 g) Cheddar cheese, grated (optional)

Wash and trim the watercress. Chop it finely and cook in the sunflower margarine for a few minutes. Then add the stock, stirring, and bring to the boil. Season with a little salt and stir in the cheese. Serve when the cheese has melted.

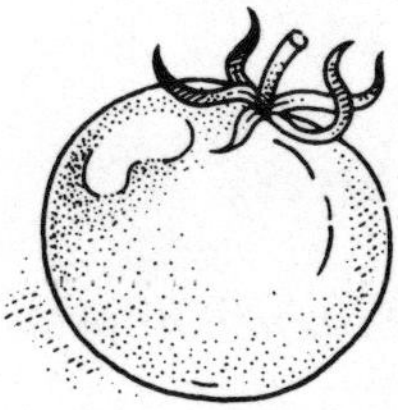

Midwinter Soup

This is a wholesome and nourishing vegetable soup to warm body and soul. A sprinkling of grated Parmesan tops it off beautifully, and I like to hand around a bowl of grated cheese and let everyone help themselves.

Makes 3 pints (1.8 litres)

12 oz (350 g) potatoes, peeled and chopped
12 oz (350 g) Brussels sprouts, trimmed and halved
1 lb (450 g) leeks, washed and chopped
3 oz (75 g) sunflower margarine
1 pint (600 ml) stock
1 pint (600 ml) milk
lemon juice
salt and pepper
freshly grated Parmesan, or other hard cheese, to serve

Sauté the prepared vegetables in the sunflower margarine, turning for 15 minutes until well softened. Add the stock and the milk and simmer until the vegetables are completely soft, about 15 minutes more. Add the lemon juice and season to taste. Blend in the food-processor until smooth, and serve with a bowl of grated cheese to hand around.

STARLIGHT SOUP Ⓒ

A thick, nourishing soup which is definitely winter food. The little star shapes look lovely dotted amongst the vegetables and it makes a hearty, satisfying lunch served simply with wholemeal bread.

Makes 2½ pints (1.4 litres)

6 oz (175 g) dried cannellini beans, soaked overnight
3 tbs olive oil
2 cloves garlic, skinned and sliced
1 small onion, chopped
3 celery sticks, trimmed and finely sliced
small bunch of parsley, chopped
14 oz (400 g) can tomatoes, chopped, juices reserved
1½ pints (900 ml) stock
salt and pepper
6 oz (175 g) stellini (tiny pasta stars)
freshly grated Parmesan cheese to serve

Drain the beans. Put into a pan, cover with fresh water and simmer for 15 minutes. Drain again.

Meanwhile heat the oil in a pan, add the garlic, onion, celery and parsley and cook gently for about 5 minutes, stirring until softened. Add the tomatoes and their juices, the stock and the beans. Cover and simmer for 1 hour or until the beans are very tender.

Scoop out about one-third of the beans and purée in a food-processor or blender, then return to the soup. Add salt and pepper to taste. Stir in the stellini and simmer for a further 8–10 minutes until they are very tender. Check the seasoning and serve sprinkled with grated Parmesan.

Secret Soup

This tasty soup is a valuable standby, since the ingredients are usually to be found on the larder shelf or vegetable rack. It's as nutritious as it is delicious.

Makes 2 pints (1.2 litres)

8 oz (250 g) can baked beans
1½ pints (900 ml) vegetable stock
4 thin slices onion
3 celery sticks, chopped
sea salt
8 oz (250 g) can tomatoes

Put the baked beans and stock in a pan with the onion and celery, bring to the boil and simmer for 10 minutes. Season with a little salt. Add the tomatoes with their juices, then pour into the food-processor and blend until smooth. Check the seasoning and it is ready to serve.

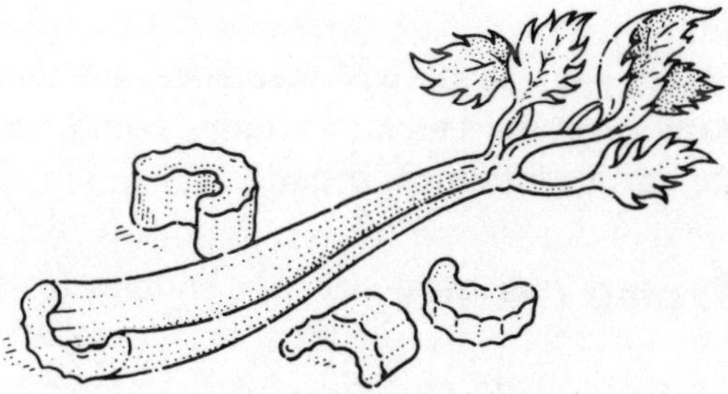

CARROT SOUP ©

So straightforward to make, and always popular with the children, this carrot soup has a wonderful golden-orange colour. Serve it at any time of the year.

Makes 1½ pints (900 ml)

8 oz (250 g) carrots, cooked (or you can use leftovers)
1 pint (600 ml) vegetable stock
¼ pint (150 ml) milk
salt and pepper

Put the carrots and stock into the food-processor and blend until smooth. Heat through and finish with a little milk. Season to taste and it is ready to serve.

You can also add to it shredded lettuce leaves, lightly sautéed in a little sunflower margarine, for a delicious summer soup.

BEAUTIFUL BEETROOT SOUP

A cold-weather soup made with beetroot and celery. The rich flavours of the vegetables make warming, comforting food. Best served with warm wholemeal bread.

Makes 1½ pints (900 ml)

1 lb (450 g) cooked beetroot, chopped
4 celery sticks, sliced
¾ pint (450 ml) stock
salt and pepper
thick yogurt or cream to finish

Put the beetroot and the celery in a saucepan, pour over the stock and simmer for 20 minutes. Blend until smooth in the food-processor. Season to taste and serve hot, stirring a tablespoon of thick yogurt or cream into each bowl of soup as you serve it.

Bread Fingers

Delicious served with any of the preceding soups.

Preheat the oven to 150°C/300°F/gas mark 2. Cut the crusts off slices of bread and cut the slices into long fingers. Spread with sunflower margarine or garlic butter (see page 151). Place on a greased baking sheet and bake for 20–30 minutes until golden and crisp.

Emergency Loaf

Handy for when the system fails and you have run out of bread. This can be made in a matter of minutes and is irresistible.

8 oz (225 g) plain flour, or 6 oz (175 g) plain and 2 oz (50 g) wholemeal flour
1 oz (25 g) sunflower margarine
1 tsp bicarbonate of soda
1 tsp cream of tartar
¼ pint (150 ml) milk

Sift the flour into a bowl and rub in the margarine. Then sift in the bicarbonate of soda and the cream of tartar. Mix quickly to a soft dough with the milk. Knead lightly until smooth. Fry in a heavy, greased pan over a moderate heat until golden-brown on both sides and cooked through – about 10 minutes altogether. Serve hot – and eat it all up, since it doesn't improve with keeping!

Quick Poppy Seed Loaf

This has been my standby for years – a yeastless bread which is made in a matter of minutes, and melts in the mouth. Use half white and half wholemeal self-raising flour if you like. If anyone objects to poppy seeds, sprinkle the dough with cracked wheat or sesame or sunflower seeds instead.

Makes 1 small loaf

8 oz (225 g) self-raising flour
1 tsp salt
¼ pint (150 ml) milk

For the topping
1 tbs milk
1 tbs water
poppy seeds

Preheat the oven to 220°C/425°F/gas mark 7. Sift the flour and salt into a large bowl, then mix quickly to a soft dough with the milk using a fork. Turn out on to a floured board and knead lightly for a minute or two until the dough is light and smooth. Shape it into a round with your hands and place it on a greased and floured baking sheet. Brush the top with a mixture of milk and water, to give it a golden crust. Sprinkle with poppy seeds and bake for 30–35 minutes. Allow to cool a little, then eat it warm. It also makes lovely nutty toast.

Lovely Lunches

The thing about lunch is that it has to happen every day – when, that is, the children are very young, or on holiday. The problem is thinking up ideas of what to give them, to provide variety. The recipes included here are relatively quick and easy to make, and provide tasty and satisfying food that children love. Many of them became the classics of my childhood, and I have adapted them to modern tastes. They seem destined to become firm favourites with the next generation.

Simplicity Chicken B

Using condensed soup as a base for sauce is fast and convenient. Alternatively use 1 pint (600 ml) Béchamel Sauce or Tomato Sauce (see pages 148–50) instead of the soup and milk. Serve with baked potatoes and vegetables.

4 chicken joints
sunflower margarine
10 oz (300 g) can condensed mushroom soup
½ pint (300 ml) milk
1 medium onion, chopped

Preheat the oven to 170°C/325°F/gas mark 3. Fry the chicken in sunflower margarine until golden-brown. Place in the bottom of an ovenproof dish. Mix the soup with the milk over a gentle heat, add the onion, then pour the mixture over the chicken pieces. Bake for 30 minutes.

Toad in the Hall

This is a kind of 'sausagemeat flan' made with light, crumbly pastry, and is very popular with the kids. You can serve it hot or cold – and it is excellent on a picnic. If using a vegetarian substitute for the sausagemeat, omit the bacon as well and fry in a little sunflower oil with the onion.

Oil Pastry (see page 153)
1 lb (450 g) sausagemeat (or use vegetarian equivalent, see above), crumbled
2 rashers bacon, chopped
1 small onion, chopped
water
salt and pepper

Line a 10 inch (25 cm) flan tin with the pastry and bake it blind (see page 153). Preheat the oven to 200°C/400°F/gas mark 6. Put the sausagemeat in a dry frying pan with the chopped bacon and onion and fry for 5 minutes, turning occasionally. Add a little water, season with salt and pepper, and simmer for 15 minutes. Put into the pastry case and cover with a lattice of pastry trimmings. Bake for 25–30 minutes or until well browned.

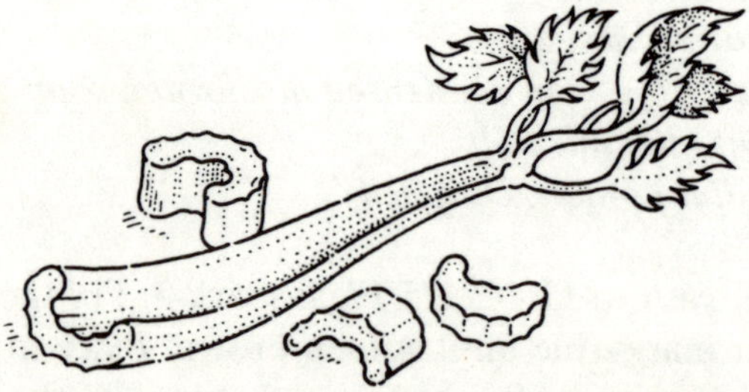

Toad's Surprise

This is extraordinarily delicious for something so easy to prepare. The sausagemeat itself is the 'flan case' which contains a simple mixture of eggs and onion. Best served with a tossed mixed salad.

12 oz (350 g) sausagemeat (or vegetarian equivalent)
1 egg
¼ pint (150 ml) milk
½ onion, chopped
salt and pepper

Preheat the oven to 190°C/375°F/gas mark 5. Line a greased 8 inch (20 cm) flan dish with the sausagemeat, pressing it out to about ¼ inch (5 mm) thick. Beat the egg with the milk, add the onion and season to taste. Pour into the case and bake for 45 minutes.

Mighty Meat Loaf

One of the simplest meat loaves in the world, this is delicious and useful family food which can be eaten hot with Tomato Sauce (see page 150) and vegetables or cold with chutney and salads.

8 oz (250 g) fresh breadcrumbs
1½ lb (750 g) lean mince (or vegetarian equivalent)
1 onion, chopped finely
salt and pepper
1 tsp celery salt
4 oz (100 g) cheese, grated
¼ pint (150 ml) tomato juice
2 large eggs

Preheat the oven to 180°C/350°F/gas mark 4. Combine all the ingredients and put into a large greased loaf tin. Bake for 1 hour. Cool in the tin on a rack for 10 minutes before attempting to turn out.

Nutty Meat Balls

These tasty meat balls are made with the addition of pounded walnuts. Deliciously different, and wonderful served with the Tomato Sauce on page 150.

2 slices wholemeal bread
milk
1 lb (450 g) lean mince (or vegetarian equivalent)
2 eggs
chopped parsley
juice and grated rind of ½ lemon
1 tbs walnuts, pounded in a mortar
salt and pepper
flour
sunflower oil

Cut the crusts off the bread and briefly soak the slices in milk. Mix all the ingredients except the flour and oil together in a bowl and season well. Shape into balls, roll in flour and fry lightly in oil. Put into a deep pan, add boiling water to cover and simmer for 20 minutes. Drain thoroughly, and serve with Tomato Sauce (see page 150).

Extraordinary Eggs

This delightful diversion into the realms of egg cookery is quick and easy to make and has a taste quite unlike the usual egg dishes. It is a wholesome meal in itself.

2 oz (50 g) bacon, chopped
2 oz (50 g) mushrooms, sliced
sunflower margarine
6 eggs, separated
salt and pepper

Crisp the bacon and fry the mushrooms in sunflower margarine, then set aside and keep warm. Pour the unbeaten egg whites into a well-greased ovenproof dish. Place over a pan of boiling water and poach them, stirring, until they begin to set. Beat the yolks, season them and pour over the whites, which should be just firm enough to support them. Keep over the heat until both yolks and whites are set. Cool slightly, run a knife around the edges and turn out. Sprinkle the bacon and mushrooms over the top, cut into wedges and serve.

Another delicious way of serving this is to cover it with a thick Onion Sauce (see page 150), coat it with grated cheese or breadcrumbs and brown it under the grill.

Potato Ring B C

A ring of golden mashed potato contains a creamy mixture of chicken garnished with chopped parsley. There are endless variations on this theme: cooked fish, mushrooms, ham, hard-boiled eggs, etc. can all take the place of chopped chicken in the sauce. Serve with favourite vegetables or a salad.

1 oz (25 g) butter
1½ lb (750 g) mashed potato
1 egg, beaten
¾ lb (350 g) cooked chicken, chopped
¾ pint (450 ml) Béchamel Sauce (see page 148)
chopped parsley

Preheat the oven to 190°C/375°F/gas mark 5. Melt the butter and mash into the potato. Form into a ring around the edge of a greased, shallow ovenproof dish 6 inches (15 cm) in diameter. Brush with beaten egg and brown in the oven for 20 minutes. Meanwhile add the chopped chicken to the sauce and heat thoroughly. Pour into the centre of the potato ring. Garnish with chopped parsley.

CHEESY POTATO BAKE C

Layers of cheese and cooked sliced potatoes are baked with milk until tender and creamy. Lovely with a tomato and onion salad, or simply as a side vegetable.

4 oz (100 g) Cheddar cheese, grated
1 lb (450 g) potatoes, cooked and sliced
2 eggs
½ pint (300 ml) milk
salt and nutmeg

Preheat the oven to 180°C/350°F/gas mark 4. Grease a baking dish and cover the base with half of the cheese. Cover evenly with the potato slices. Mix together the eggs, milk and seasonings and pour over the top. Cover with the rest of the cheese and bake for 45 minutes.

NICE AND CHEESY RICE B C

A wholesome and nourishing country recipe which is excellent fuel for hungry kids! Serve it with salad, or lightly steamed vegetables.

6 oz (175 g) rice
4 eggs, separated
1 pint (600 ml) milk
1 oz (25 g) sunflower margarine, melted
4 oz (100 g) Cheddar cheese, grated
salt and pepper

Preheat the oven to 180°C/350°F/gas mark 4. Cook the rice. Beat the egg yolks and add them to the cooked rice with the milk, sunflower margarine and cheese. Season with salt and pepper.

Beat the egg whites until they are very stiff, then fold into the rice mixture. Bake in a greased ovenproof dish for 25 minutes.

CRUSTY CHEESE Ⓒ

A golden crust of bread encases a rich, creamy cheese filling. Cold-weather food, lovely with baked potatoes.

4 slices day-old bread
sunflower margarine
2 eggs, beaten
½ pint (300 ml) single cream
½ tsp mustard powder
6 oz (175 g) Cheddar cheese, cut into small dice
salt and pepper

Preheat the oven to 180°C/350°F/gas mark 4. Cut the crusts off the bread, spread the slices with sunflower margarine and cut each slice into 8 strips. Put a layer in a greased baking dish and arrange the rest of the strips upright around the sides. Mix together the remaining ingredients and pour into the centre. Bake for 30 minutes.

LITTLE SOUFFLÉ FLANS

These light little flans are made with crumbly oil pastry and a soufflé-type filling. Great weekend food, delicious with lightly steamed courgettes and a side salad.

Oil Pastry (see page 153)

For the filling
¼ pint (150 ml) milk
2 oz (50 g) fresh granary breadcrumbs
1 oz (25 g) sunflower margarine
4 oz (100 g) Cheddar cheese, grated, or 3 oz (75 g) sweetcorn
1 egg, separated
salt, pepper and mustard

Bring the milk to the boil, stir in the breadcrumbs and sunflower margarine, and leave to cool.

Preheat the oven to 190°C/375°F/gas mark 5. Line some little greased patty-tins with the pastry, pressed out thinly. Sprinkle a little of the cheese in the bottom of each. Beat the egg yolk and add to the breadcrumb mixture with the rest of the cheese and seasonings. Beat the egg white stiffly and fold into the mixture. Turn into the pastry cases and bake for 20–30 minutes. Cool a little, then lift out carefully and serve.

Lip-Licking Ways with Vegetables

There are all sorts of ways to make vegetables more attractive to young eaters. If yours turn their noses up at plainly cooked vegetables, try serving them up in Béchamel Sauce (see page 148). Carrots, marrow, cauliflower, broad beans, leeks and even beetroot all take on a new attraction when coated in a creamy sauce. You may also find that children will happily eat mashed or puréed vegetables that they stubbornly refuse to eat in any other form. Add a little butter or cream to the purée and season to taste.

Lettuce

Cut a lettuce heart into quarters and cook in a little butter over a low heat, closely covered. Shake frequently, then season with salt and pepper and chopped fresh herbs. Particularly good with Welsh Rarebit (see page 91).

Peas

Ever tried cooking frozen peas straight from the freezer in a little sunflower margarine? Toss them until they are heated through but still crisp: they are wonderful.

Cabbage

Deep-fry finely shredded leftover cooked cabbage in hot vegetable oil until crisp. It is simply delectable.

Beansprouts

Stir-fry lightly in sunflower margarine or oil until they are hot through but still crisp.

Potatoes

Thinly slice raw potatoes and sauté them in butter, turning constantly, until the slices are coated. Then leave to cook, covered, over a gentle heat until the bottom is browned and the rest cooked through.

Carrots B C

How about trying this out on a child who emphatically declares that he hates carrots: a mixture of potatoes and carrots cooked together and mashed with sunflower margarine and milk?

CREAMY CARROTS C

A delicious way of cooking carrots for choosy kids. Serve as a side vegetable with roast chicken and baked potatoes.

4 spring onions, chopped
1½ oz (40 g) sunflower margarine
10–12 small carrots, washed
salt and pepper
chopped parsley
¼ pint (150 ml) single cream

Preheat the oven to 180°C/350°F/gas mark 4. Fry the chopped onions in the sunflower margarine over a gentle heat until soft. Put into an ovenproof dish with the whole carrots, seasonings and parsley. Pour the cream over the top and bake, covered with foil, for 45 minutes.

FRIED CABBAGE AND NUTS

One of the best ways I have yet discovered of getting children to enjoy their greens!

olive oil
½ medium onion, thinly sliced and shredded
1 medium cabbage (or try it with 1 medium cauliflower, 1 crisp lettuce, 12 oz/350 g spring greens etc.), finely shredded
2 oz (50 g) mixed walnuts and raw peanuts, chopped
salt and pepper

Heat some olive oil in a heavy pan. Place the onion and cabbage in the pan with the chopped nuts. Cover and cook very gently for 10–15 minutes, stirring occasionally. Season with salt and pepper, and serve.

☆ Salad Spectaculars ☆

The secret of preparing salads for kids is to fill them with tasty morsels of their favourite things – in my experience kids are very selective about salads! So here are some ideas for tempting the little monsters into eating 'raw food'. Remember that appearance is everything and if you tempt the eye you'll more than likely tempt the palate too. Ring the changes by colouring mayonnaise pink with a little tomato ketchup, or give it a speckled look with the addition of chopped fresh herbs or watercress. I like to mix mayonnaise half and half with plain low-fat yogurt to make a healthier dressing.

- Banana slices, nut, orange wedges and lettuce, with mayonnaise.
- Orange sections, tomato wedges, chopped celery and peanuts in light mayonnaise.

- Pineapple chunks, cottage cheese, chopped celery and nuts mixed with a little mayonnaise.
- Chunks of banana rolled in finely chopped peanuts or walnuts and serve on dressed lettuce.
- Tuna, chopped celery and tomato wedges dressed with mayonnaise.
- Cold diced turkey with peas, celery, walnuts and mayonnaise, served on lettuce.
- Sardines, hard-boiled eggs, tomatoes and mayonnaise.
- Cold cooked pasta mixed with finely chopped raw vegetables and tossed in vinaigrette.
- Chopped cooked potato and hard-boiled egg quarters in vinaigrette.
- Peeled, grated cucumber dressed in vinaigrette or mayonnaise.

TOADSTOOLS

The effect of these toadstools is very charming for a special salad – slightly time-consuming to prepare, but they make a memorable meal.

4 hard-boiled eggs
¼ pint (150 ml) cooked shrimps, finely chopped
2 tbs Mayonnaise (see page 151)
2 lettuce leaves
2 small tomatoes

Cut a slice from the blunt end of each egg and set aside. Remove the yolks, leaving the whites whole. Cut a slice off the other end so that the eggs can stand up. Mash the yolks with a fork, then mix together with the finely chopped shrimps and the mayonnaise. Stuff each egg with one quarter of the mixture and place on a lettuce leaf. Cut the tomatoes in half, scoop out the centres and place upside down on top of each egg. Chop leftover egg whites and decorate the tomato tops.

Funny Bunny Salad

Put half a canned or peeled and cored fresh pear, rounded side up, on a bed of shredded lettuce and cottage cheese. Insert almonds for ears, and carrot rings for eyes and nose. Use a tiny button mushroom for the tail.

☆ Perfect Pasta ☆

Pasta is generally a great success with children – they seem to love it, and it is easy to make it the basis of a healthy and balanced meal. Perfect for lunch or supper, depending on the programme of the day, these recipes give you a wide variety of ideas – no doubt the kids will decide which ones are their favourites! You can delight them with all the various shapes – from twists to bows and from ribbons to macaroni. It comes in different colours too and you can try mixing white spaghetti with green, for example, to make a colourful change. When they grow up into teenagers, pasta dishes are among the first things your kids are likely to make for themselves, since they are so simple and rewarding.

Nutty Pasta with Cauliflower

This delightful golden dish is a light, dry mixture of cauliflower florets spiced with saffron and tarragon – for more sophisticated kids, perhaps. Browned pine nuts add their crunch to this winning combination.

1 tsp saffron threads
2 tbs stock
½ cauliflower, cut into tiny florets
1 tbs chopped tarragon
1 oz (25 g) pine nuts, browned under the grill
12 oz (350 g) pasta bows
2 tbs olive oil
salt and pepper

Soak the saffron in the stock. Steam the cauliflower florets for 5 minutes or until tender, then put in a bowl with the tarragon, and add the saffron stock and pine nuts. Meanwhile cook the pasta bows 'al dente'.

Toss the hot, drained pasta in the olive oil, then combine thoroughly with the cauliflower mixture. Season to taste.

Tagliatelle with Vegetables and Crispy Bacon

A popular family dish which is simple to prepare.

2 tbs olive oil
2 tbs chopped onion
4 oz (100 g) bacon, diced
8 oz (225 g) small button mushrooms, sliced
8 oz (225 g) peas, cooked
salt and pepper
12 oz (350 g) tagliatelle
freshly grated Parmesan cheese to serve

Heat the oil in a pan, add the onion and bacon and fry for about 5 minutes until the bacon is slightly crisp and the onion lightly browned. Add the mushrooms, stir until well coated and cook for a few minutes until they just begin to soften. Add the peas, mix well and heat through. Season with salt and pepper. Meanwhile cook the tagliatelle 'al dente'.

Add the vegetable mixture to the hot, drained tagliatelle and toss well. Serve immediately, sprinkled with Parmesan.

Pasta Bows with Broccoli and Creamy Mushroom Sauce

Broccoli florets go beautifully with tiny pasta bows and this delicate sauce, a creamy purée of mushrooms, is spooned over the dish to moisten and flavour it. Serve it with a crisp, tossed salad and warm granary rolls.

2 oz (50 g) sunflower margarine
1 tbs flour
4 fl oz (120 ml) milk
salt and pepper
8 oz (225 g) mushrooms, chopped roughly
¼ pint (150 ml) single cream
1 lb (450 g) broccoli florets
2 tbs olive oil
6 spring onions, trimmed and sliced finely
12 oz (350 g) tiny pasta bows

For the mushroom sauce, melt 1 oz (25 g) of the sunflower margarine in a pan and stir in the flour until smooth. Gradually add the milk, stirring until the sauce thickens, then add salt and pepper to taste and simmer gently for 5 minutes, stirring. Heat the remaining sunflower margarine, add the mushrooms and cook for about 5 minutes until softened and cooked down, stirring all the time. Add the cream and simmer gently for 5 minutes, stirring. Season to taste. Stir in the white sauce and purée in the food-processor or blender. Heat through before serving.

Steam the broccoli for 3–4 minutes. Heat the oil in a pan, add the spring onions and fry gently for 3–4 minutes, stirring until softened. Add the broccoli and stir-fry until coated with the oil and well mixed with the spring onions. Meanwhile cook the pasta bows 'al dente'.

Add the stir-fried vegetables to the hot, drained pasta bows and toss well. Serve on warm plates, with the mushroom sauce spooned over the top.

TASTY TUNA [B]

I have made this spaghetti dish countless times for my hungry children and it has become a firm favourite. The great bonus is that the dish takes no time to prepare and is a meal in itself.

7 oz (200 g) can tuna
2 tbs olive oil
34 tbs chopped fresh parsley
4 fl oz (120 ml) vegetable stock
pepper
12 oz (350 g) spaghetti

Drain and flake the tuna. Heat the olive oil in a pan, add the tuna and parsley and toss for 5 minutes. Pour in the stock and heat through. Simmer for 5 minutes, then add plenty of pepper. Meanwhile cook the spaghetti 'al dente'.

Add the sauce to the hot, drained spaghetti and toss well.

TUNA NOODLE DOODLE [C]

This recipe has endless variations. You can use chopped chicken instead of fish; Mushroom Sauce (see page 149), Béchamel Sauce (see page 148), or thick Tomato Sauce (see page 150) instead of the soup.

8 oz (250 g) noodles, cooked
7 oz (200 g) can tuna
10 oz (300 g) can condensed mushroom soup
¼ pint (150 ml) milk
4 oz (100 g) frozen peas or leftover Brussels sprouts
salt and pepper
4 tbs dried breadcrumbs

Preheat the oven to 170°C/325°F/gas mark 3. Mix the first five ingredients together, season, and put into a greased ovenproof dish. Sprinkle with breadcrumbs. Bake for 30 minutes.

Zippy Fish

Food for all the family, and much loved by the kids. Pasta is mixed with tasty vegetables and white fish, and baked with cheese. Serve with a simple green salad.

8 oz (250 g) pasta shells
4 oz (100 g) celery, chopped
a little green pepper, chopped (optional)
1 lb (450 g) can tomatoes
1 tsp soy sauce
12 oz (350 g) cod or haddock, cooked and flaked
salt and pepper
2 oz (50 g) cheese, grated

Preheat the oven to 180°C/350°F/gas mark 4. Cook the pasta in boiling, salted water for 7–8 minutes, or until 'al dente'. Combine the rest of the ingredients except the cheese and fold into the pasta. Season to taste. Pour the mixture into a greased ovenproof dish, sprinkle the cheese over the top, and bake for 25 minutes.

Cock a Doodle Noodles

Scrumptious layers of cheesy noodles and chicken are topped with a mild mustard sauce. A winner.

8 oz (250 g) egg noodles
1½ oz (40 g) cheese, grated
1 lb (450 g) cooked chicken, sliced
¾ pint (450 ml) Mild Mustard Sauce *(see page 149)*

Preheat the oven to 190°C/375°F/gas mark 5. Cook the noodles 'al dente'. Drain, and stir in the cheese. Season and put in greased ovenproof dish. Cover with the pieces of chicken and pour the sauce over the top. Bake for 20–30 minutes until well browned.

CHICKEN IN THE STRAW AND HAY

'Straw and hay' is the local Italian name for the combination of yellow and green noodles in this amusing dish. Its subtle colours are highlighted by the greens of mange-tout and petits pois, which also add crunch and flavour to this chicken and pasta recipe.

2 tbs olive oil
2 shallots, finely sliced
4 oz (100 g) mange-tout
4 oz (100 g) petits pois
8 oz (225 g) chicken breast meat, sliced
¼ pint (150 ml) white wine
¼ pint (150 ml) stock
salt and pepper
6 oz (175 g) yellow tagliatelle
6 oz (175 g) tagliatelle verde
1 egg, beaten
freshly grated Parmesan cheese to serve

Heat the oil in a pan, add the shallots and fry gently for 3–4 minutes until softened. Add the mange-tout and petits pois and stir-fry for 3 minutes until they begin to soften. Stir in the chicken slices and pour in the white wine and stock. Heat through, stirring, and simmer for 5 minutes until the chicken is cooked and the sauce reduces a little. Add salt and pepper to taste. Meanwhile cook the tagliatelle 'al dente'.

Toss the hot, drained tagliatelle in a pan with the chicken and vegetables, mix in the beaten egg and shake over a gentle heat until lightly set. Serve at once with grated cheese.

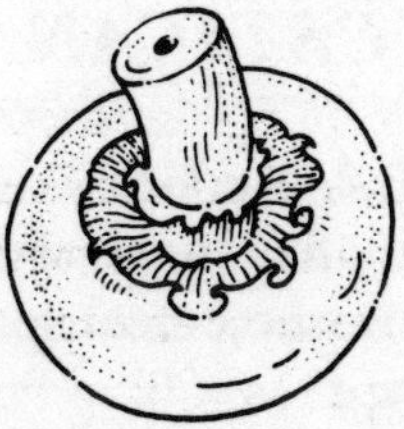

EGGS IN A CHICKEN'S NEST Ⓒ

One of my kids' favourite winter supper dishes, this luscious concoction makes a warming and satisfying meal. Soft-boiled eggs nestle in a ring of macaroni which has been tossed in a creamy mixture of chicken, garlic and mushrooms.

4 large eggs
2 oz (50 g) sunflower margarine
1 clove garlic, skinned and sliced finely
4 oz (100 g) mushrooms, sliced
6 oz (175 g) cooked chicken meat, diced
¼ pint (150 ml) single cream
salt and pepper
12 oz (350 g) macaroni
freshly grated Parmesan cheese to serve

Plunge the eggs carefully into a pan of boiling water and simmer for 4 minutes exactly, then plunge into cold water for 2 minutes. Peel gently and keep the eggs warm.

Melt the sunflower margarine in a pan, add the garlic and fry gently for 5 minutes until softened. Stir in the mushrooms and chicken and toss until the mushrooms are cooked but still crisp. Add the cream and heat through. Season with salt and pepper to taste. Meanwhile cook the macaroni 'al dente'. Stir the creamy chicken mixture into the hot, drained macaroni.

Line a warmed round serving dish with the macaroni and place the eggs in the middle. Serve with grated Parmesan.

SPAGHETTI RUSTICANA

This tomato sauce is an Italian country recipe and has deservedly become a classic. Lightly flavoured with basil and oregano, it goes especially well with wholemeal spaghetti, but you can of course use any pasta shapes you like. Perfect family food.

3–4 tbs olive oil
4 medium onions, chopped finely
2 lb (900 g) tomatoes, skinned (or two 14 oz/400 g cans tomatoes, drained)
2 cloves garlic, skinned and chopped very finely
1 bay leaf
1 tbs chopped fresh oregano
1 tbs chopped fresh basil
salt and pepper
1 lb (450 g) spaghetti
freshly grated Parmesan cheese to serve

Heat the olive oil in a pan, add the onions, cover and cook very gently for about 12 minutes, stirring from time to time until very soft and slightly sweet. Add the tomatoes, garlic and bay leaf and mix thoroughly. Cook, uncovered, over a low heat for 25–30 minutes. Remove the bay leaf, add the chopped herbs and salt and pepper to taste. Meanwhile cook the spaghetti 'al dente'.

Serve the hot, drained spaghetti with the sauce spooned over each helping. Hand around grated Parmesan to sprinkle over the top.

Cockaleekie Pasta Twists

Leeks go especially well with chicken, and mixed into pasta twists make a perfect dish. Hand around grated Parmesan and a pepper mill for everyone to help themselves.

3 oz (75 g) sunflower margarine
2 lb (900 g) leeks, washed and sliced finely
4 fl oz (120 ml) chicken stock
8 oz (225 g) cooked chicken meat, cut into small cubes
salt and pepper
12 oz (350 g) pasta twists
freshly grated Parmesan cheese to serve

Melt the sunflower margarine in a pan, add the leeks and fry gently for 10 minutes, stirring from time to time until completely soft. Stir in the stock and simmer for a further 10 minutes. Finally stir in the chicken, heat through and add salt and pepper to taste. Meanwhile cook the pasta twists 'al dente'.

Mix the chicken and leeks into the hot, drained pasta, toss thoroughly and serve with grated Parmesan.

Henny Penne

Adding watercress to a combination of chicken and pasta makes an elegant and tasty dish. It is then coated with cheese and breadcrumbs and browned lightly.

2 tbs olive oil
4 oz (100 g) mushrooms, sliced
1 clove garlic, skinned and crushed
4 spring onions, trimmed and sliced
8 oz (225 g) cooked chicken meat, shredded
salt and pepper
¼ pint (150 ml) chicken stock
1 bunch watercress, trimmed and chopped very finely
12 oz (350 g) penne
2 oz (50 g) cheese, grated
2 tbs dried breadcrumbs

Heat the oil in a pan, add the mushrooms and fry for 3 minutes until cooked through but still crisp. Add the garlic and spring onions and toss together for 1–2 minutes. Stir in the chicken, heat through and add salt and pepper to taste. Add the stock and bring to simmering point. Stir in the watercress and cook gently for 3–4 minutes. Check the seasoning. Meanwhile cook the penne 'al dente'.

Toss the chicken and sauce into the hot, drained penne and transfer to a warmed flameproof serving dish. Combine the cheese and breadcrumbs and sprinkle over the top. Brown under the grill briefly, and serve piping hot.

Pasta Bows with Flageolets

The versatility of this dish is amazing. You can eat it hot, sprinkled with grated Parmesan. Or try it warm, with lightly steamed vegetables. Cold, as salad, it makes a lovely summery lunch.

8 oz (225 g) pasta bows
14 oz (400 g) can flageolet beans
4–5 tbs pesto sauce
fresh basil leaves to garnish

Cook the pasta bows 'al dente'. Meanwhile heat the flageolets with their juices from the can over a gentle heat. When hot, drain and toss into the hot, drained pasta bows. Stir in the pesto and mix thoroughly. Garnish with basil leaves.

Noodle Custards Ⓒ

Serve this mouth-wateringly soft dish of lightly set, savoury egg custard and noodles with crisply steamed broccoli and granary bread.

2 oz (50 g) bean-thread noodles
1 chicken breast, cooked and shredded
3 oz (75 g) peas
4 oz (100 g) mange-tout, trimmed and sliced
6 spring onions, trimmed and sliced finely
1–2 tbs soy sauce
½ pint (300 ml) stock
6 eggs, beaten

Preheat the oven to 180°C/350°F/gas mark 4. Soak the noodles in hot water for 10 minutes, then drain. Mix the chicken, noodles, peas, mange-tout and spring onions together and add soy sauce to taste. Put into four individual ovenproof dishes.

Mix the stock into the beaten eggs and divide among the dishes, then bake for about 15 minutes until lightly set. Leave to cool a little and serve warm.

Pasta Shells in a Chinese Sauce

A gorgeous and unusual dish which makes a delightful change from more western ideas of cooking pasta. Adventurous kids love it.

6 oz (175 g) beansprouts
6 oz (175 g) water chestnuts, slivered
4 oz (100 g) small button mushrooms, halved
4 oz (100 g) lychees, stoned and sliced
1 inch (2.5 cm) fresh root ginger, peeled and grated
2 cloves garlic, skinned and crushed
2 tbs soy sauce
2 tbs raspberry vinegar
8 oz (225 g) pasta shells
2 tbs sesame oil

Mix the beansprouts, water chestnuts, mushrooms and lychees together. Stir the ginger and garlic into the soy sauce then add the raspberry vinegar. Cook the pasta shells 'al dente'.

Toss the warm, drained pasta shells in the sesame oil, then combine with the vegetable and fruit mixture. Toss the salad in the spiced dressing. Serve at room temperature.

Spaghetti Carbonara

This classic Italian dish is a soft, creamy mixture of lightly set eggs, with ham and basil as the predominant flavours. It makes a quick and luscious lunch, accompanied by a crisp, tossed salad and hot garlic bread.

12 oz (350 g) spaghetti
1 oz (25 g) sunflower margarine
4 oz (100 g) ham, sliced and cut into thin strips
2 tbs chopped fresh basil
3 eggs, beaten
pepper
freshly grated Parmesan cheese to serve

Cook the spaghetti until 'al dente'. Meanwhile, melt the sunflower margarine in a large pan, add the ham strips and cook gently for 3–4 minutes, stirring, until heated through. Add the basil and cook for 1 minute.

Add the cooked, drained spaghetti to the pan. Stir in the beaten eggs and cook over a low heat as for scrambled eggs, stirring constantly. Add plenty of pepper. Serve immediately, with grated Parmesan to hand around.

Rodeo Spaghetti

Serve this tasty version of spaghetti bolognese with a tossed salad to make a perfect meal for all the family.

2 onions, sliced
sunflower margarine
1 lb (450 g) lean mince (or vegetarian substitute)
¾ pint (450 ml) Tomato Sauce (see page 150)
4 oz (100 g) mushrooms
8 oz (225 g) pasta shapes
salt and pepper
grated cheese to serve (optional)

Fry the onions gently in the sunflower margarine. Increase the heat slightly, add the mince and fry until browned, turning all the time Add the tomato sauce and the mushrooms and simmer for 15 minutes. Season well.

Meanwhile cook the pasta 'al dente'. Mix the sauce into the pasta and serve hot, with grated cheese if liked.

Mushroom Fettucine Ⓒ

This is a rich dish, so a little goes a long way. The creamy sauce with mushrooms and ham is enriched with eggs, cooked until lightly set. A green salad on the side is the ideal accompaniment.

2 tbs olive oil
1 Spanish onion, chopped finely
6 oz (175 g) mushrooms, sliced
4 oz (100 g) ham, diced
¼ pint (150 ml) single cream
2 eggs, beaten
salt and pepper
12 oz (350 g) fettucine
freshly grated Parmesan cheese to serve

Heat the oil in a pan, add the onion and fry gently for about 5 minutes until softened. Add the mushrooms and ham and cook for about 3 minutes until the mushrooms are soft. Stir the cream into the beaten eggs and add salt and pepper to taste. Add to the mixture in the pan and cook gently until it begins to thicken, stirring all the time. Check the seasoning. Meanwhile cook the fettucine 'al dente'.

Toss the cream mixture into the hot, drained fettucine. Serve with grated Parmesan.

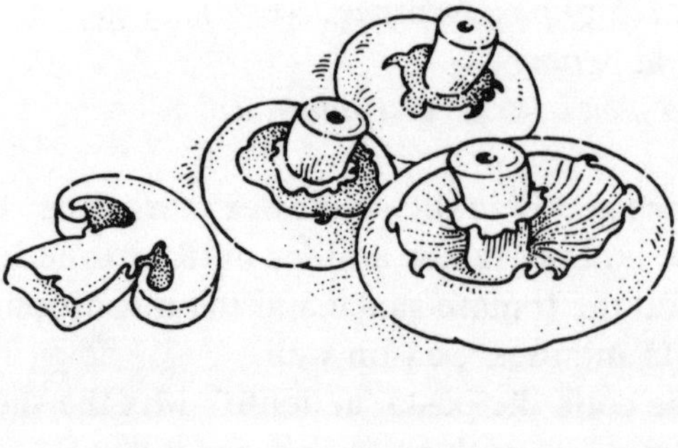

Vegetable Lasagne

Making lasagne with 'no pre-cook' pasta is the easiest thing in the world. This family recipe uses canned vegetables and is made in no time at all – and of course you can vary the ingredients. It is very popular – truly satisfying food which is a meal in itself.

14 oz (400 g) can tomatoes
salt and pepper
mixed dried herbs
2 tbs oil
6 oz (175 g) mushrooms, sliced
1 pint (600 ml) Béchamel Sauce (see page 148)
two 8 oz (225 g) cans spinach, drained
14 oz (400 g) can sweetcorn, drained
6 oz (175 g) 'no pre-cook' lasagne sheets
½ pint (300 ml) Mild Mustard Sauce (see page 149)

Preheat the oven to 180°C/350°F/gas mark 4. Drain and chop the tomatoes. Add salt, pepper and herbs to taste. Set aside. Heat the oil in a pan, add the mushrooms and fry quickly for 2 minutes until cooked but still crisp.

Divide the béchamel sauce into four. Mix the mushrooms with a quarter of the béchamel sauce. Stir the spinach into another quarter and stir the sweetcorn into the remaining two quarters of the sauce. Check the seasoning of all three fillings.

Make layers of the tomato mixture and the béchamel sauce mixtures between layers of lasagne sheets. Cover with the mild mustard sauce and bake for 45–50 minutes.

LEEKY PASTA SOUFFLÉ

The good thing about this soufflé is not only its tempting tastes – leeks, Gruyère and pasta are an incomparable combination – but the fact that it does not sink dramatically when you take it out of the oven! It is more substantial than a soufflé made with eggs alone. You can also try it with tomatoes instead of leeks.

4 oz (100 g) tagliatelle, cooked 'al dente'
¼ pint (150 ml) Béchamel Sauce (see page 148)
3 oz (75 g) Gruyère cheese, grated
salt and pepper
8 oz (225 g) leeks, washed and sliced finely
2 eggs, separated

Preheat the oven to 180°C/350°F/gas mark 4. Drain and chop the tagliatelle. Mix into the béchamel sauce with the cheese and add salt and pepper to taste.

Steam the leeks for about 8–10 minutes until tender. Beat the egg yolks well, then mix the leeks and egg yolks into the sauce. Whisk the egg whites until very stiff, then fold into the mixture.

Pour into a well-greased soufflé dish and bake for 30–35 minutes until risen and lightly set in the centre. Serve immediately.

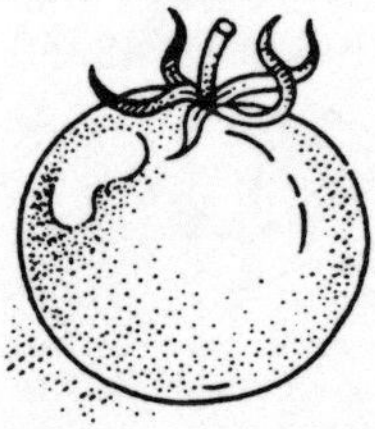

Pink Pasta Omelette

For a quick and delicious meal, this has no peer – lovely soft textures, the aroma of fresh herbs and the mouth-watering addition of cooked vermicelli. A garnish of mushrooms makes it a more complete dish, and all it needs to go with it is warm, crusty granary bread.

Serves 2

2 canned tomatoes, chopped very finely
1 tbs finely chopped fresh herbs
3 eggs, beaten
salt and pepper
4 oz (100 g) vermicelli, cooked
1½ oz (40 g) sunflower margarine
4 oz (100 g) mushrooms, sliced
small bunch of watercress, trimmed

Mix the chopped tomatoes and herbs into the beaten eggs and add salt and pepper to taste. Chop the vermicelli and fold into the egg mixture. Heat half of the sunflower margarine in a large, heavy, shallow pan and cook the omelette in the usual way.

Meanwhile heat the remaining sunflower margarine in another pan and fry the mushrooms for the garnish. Serve the omelette surrounded by the mushrooms and watercress.

Cosy Suppers

Supper can be made into a special occasion, a celebration at the end of the day when the family are around the table together for perhaps the only time. In winter, my kids love to eat by candlelight, which makes a memorable occasion of it, and throws defiance at the long grey days of the season. At any time of the year, however, these recipes provide simple yet satisfying family food to send the kids contentedly to bed. The end of another cooking day at last . . .

Cauliflower Gratinata 🄱 🄲

Lovely wholesome, nourishing food for tired children at the end of the day.

6 oz (175 g) macaroni
1 large cauliflower
¾ pint (450 ml) Béchamel Sauce (see page 148)
4 oz (100 g) Cheddar cheese, grated
4 tomatoes, sliced
extra grated cheese

Preheat the oven to 220°C/425°F/gas mark 7. Cook the macaroni 'al dente'. Steam the cauliflower until tender, then drain and cut it into florets. Add the cheese to the béchamel sauce. Combine half the sauce with the macaroni and place it on the bottom of a greased baking dish. Arrange the tomato slices around the edge of the dish and pile the cauliflower in the centre. Spoon over the rest of the sauce. Top with more cheese and bake for 30 minutes. Serve hot.

Lazy Fish Layers B C

Easy to cook and not very difficult to eat either – simple layers of fresh fish in a cream sauce with breadcrumbs and hard-boiled eggs.

4 oz (100 g) breadcrumbs, toasted
1 lb (450 g) cooked cod, mackerel or skate
1 pint (600 ml) Sauce à la Crème (see page 149)
3 hard-boiled eggs, sliced

Preheat the oven to 190°C/375°F/gas mark 5. Grease an ovenproof dish and line with half of the breadcrumbs. Add the fish to the sauce and make alternate layers with the fish mixture and the sliced eggs. Cover with the rest of the breadcrumbs and bake for about 20–25 minutes until the top is brown.

Igloo Fish B C

A light supper dish which consists of fresh fish in a white sauce, covered with a layer of soufflé. Candlelight food.

1/4 pint (150 ml) Béchamel Sauce (see page 148)
8 oz (225 g) cooked fish, flaked
3 egg whites
1 1/2 oz (40 g) Parmesan cheese, finely grated

Preheat the oven to 230°C/450°F/gas mark 8. Heat the béchamel sauce and mix with the fish. Put in the bottom of a soufflé dish. Beat the egg whites until stiff, then fold in the cheese. Spread over the fish and bake for about 10 minutes, until browned.

Funtime Fish Flan

This cold flan makes a perfect supper for a summer's evening.

Oil Pastry (see page 153)
1 lb (450 g) cooked cod or hake, flaked
¼ pint (150 ml) mayonnaise
a few gherkins, mushrooms and tomatoes

Line a 10 inch (25 cm) flan dish with oil pastry and bake blind (see page 153). Mix the fish with the mayonnaise. Chop the gherkins finely and slice the mushrooms and tomatoes thinly. Stir the gherkins and mushrooms into the fish mixture, put into the pastry case and decorate with thinly sliced tomatoes.

Toads in Cheesy Holes

So much tastier than their ordinary holes! The sausages are cooked in a cheesy batter which turns deep golden-brown.

1½ lb (750 g) chipolata sausages (or vegetarian equivalent)

For the batter
2 eggs
4 oz (100 g) plain flour, sifted
½ tsp salt
¾ pint (450 ml) milk and water mixed
3 oz (75 g) Cheddar cheese, grated

Preheat the oven to 200°C/400°F/gas mark 6. To make the batter, beat the eggs well, then stir in the sifted flour and salt. Gradually stir in the liquid until the batter becomes creamy, then add the cheese.

Fry or grill the sausages until they are well browned, then put them in a shallow, greased, ovenproof dish. Pour the batter over and bake for 30–35 minutes, until crisp and golden.

MOLE IN THE HOLE

A variation on Toad in the Hole, this uses meatballs – or vegetarian equivalent – instead of sausages. Lovely with fresh-tasting Tomato Sauce (see page 150).

Make the batter as for the Toads above, and pour over Nutty Meat Balls (see page 30) in a shallow ovenproof dish. Bake as above.

ROLY POLY PANCAKES

A simple supper dish, for a light meal with steamed vegetables.

Roll up a slice of ham in a Pancake (see page 152) and warm through in a moderate oven. Make a Béchamel Sauce (see page 148) and add mustard to taste, and a little cream. Pour over the pancake just before serving.

HAM AND POTATO BAKE [B] [C]

Family food, this is made up of layers of potato, onion and ham baked slowly until all the flavours and textures mingle.

4 potatoes, peeled and sliced
1 onion, sliced
6 oz (175 g) cooked ham, sliced
salt and pepper
milk
sunflower margarine

Preheat the oven to 180°C/350°F/gas mark 4. Grease an ovenproof dish and make alternate layers of potato, onion and ham, seasoning each layer with salt and pepper as you go. Repeat until the dish is full. Pour in milk until the dish is three-quarters full, dot with sunflower margarine and bake for 1½ hours.

CARROT CRATER Ⓒ

The centre of this ring-mould of mashed carrot can be filled with almost anything you like. Try creamed peas, pieces of cooked chicken, ham or fish – your choice.

1 lb (450 g) carrots, cooked and mashed
2 tsp grated onion
1 oz (25 g) sunflower margarine, melted
2 eggs, well beaten
1 tbs flour
¼ pint (150 ml) top of the milk or single cream
1 oz (25 g) fresh breadcrumbs
salt and pepper

Preheat the oven to 180°C/350°F/gas mark 4. Mix all the ingredients and put into a greased ring-mould. Bake for 20–30 minutes or until set.

CHICKEN ROLL

A brilliant supper dish. Serve this light, aromatic 'Swiss roll' of chicken with the Mushroom Sauce on page 149 or the Tomato Sauce on page 150.

8 oz (225 g) cooked chicken meat, chopped
½ onion, chopped finely
a little Béchamel Sauce (see page 148) or single cream
salt and pepper
6 oz (175 g) Little Miss Muffin dough made with 6 oz (175 g) flour in total (see page 120)

Mix the chicken and onion with enough béchamel or cream to moisten, and season to taste. Roll out the dough into a rectangle and put the mixture in the middle. Wet the edges and roll it up. Seal the ends securely and place with the fold underneath in a greased ovenproof dish or baking tray. Bake for 20–30 minutes or until well browned. Cut into slices and serve.

CHUCKLING CHICKEN

Chicken breasts coated in cheese and fried until tender, served on a bed of rice with tomatoes and mushrooms. It's a complete meal in itself.

4 boned chicken breasts
lemon juice
olive oil
3 tbs flour, seasoned with salt and pepper
2 oz (50 g) Parmesan cheese, grated
sunflower margarine
8 oz (225 g) rice
knob of butter
2 tomatoes, sliced
4 oz (100 g) button mushrooms

Sprinkle the chicken breasts with lemon juice and oil and leave to marinate for a while. Coat the chicken pieces with the seasoned flour and roll in the Parmesan to make quite a thick coating. Fry them in sunflower margarine, turning until the chicken is cooked.

Meanwhile cook the rice and butter it lightly. Fry the sliced tomatoes and the mushrooms in a little margarine.

Place the rice in a shallow dish and arrange the chicken around the edge. Put the fried tomatoes and mushrooms in the middle, and serve.

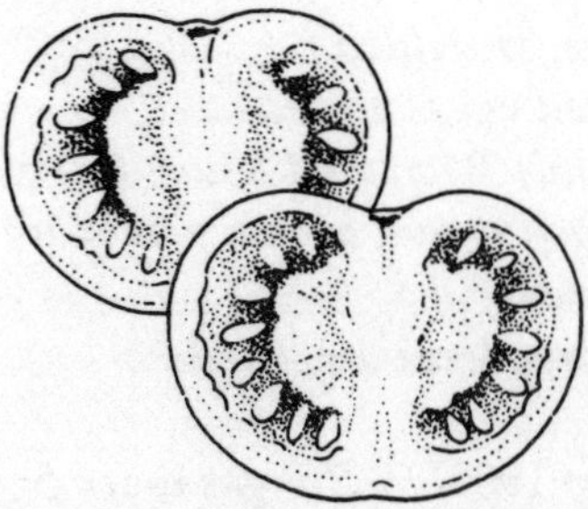

CHEDDAR FONDUE

Family food *par excellence*. Time to light the candles and start dipping the fondue forks into the pot.

2–3 tbs cornflour
1 tsp dry mustard
pepper
½ pint (300 ml) dry cider
1 oz (25 g) sunflower margarine
1 lb (450 g) Cheddar cheese, grated
fresh vegetables, sliced
bread, cut into small cubes

Blend the cornflour, mustard and pepper to a smooth cream with a little of the cider and set aside. Melt the sunflower margarine in a fondue pot, then add the cheese and the remaining cider. Heat gently and stir until smooth. Add the flour mixture, turn the heat up a little and stir until it thickens. Let it bubble gently while you dip in – using fondue forks – slices of raw celery, carrot, mushroom, cucumber, and small cubes of fresh bread.

JIVING EGGS Ⓒ

This rather unusual recipe is actually very tasty indeed and always proves popular. My kids adore it!

1 crisp lettuce, shredded
4–5 soft-boiled eggs, halved
¾ pint (450 ml) Béchamel Sauce (see page 148), made with as much cream as you can spare
chopped chives
2 oz (50 g) breadcrumbs, fried

Preheat the oven to 190°C/375°F/gas mark 5. Cover the

bottom of a greased ovenproof dish with the shredded lettuce. Place the eggs over the lettuce. Add masses of chopped chives to the béchamel sauce and pour over the top. Bake for 10–15 minutes. Serve sprinkled with fried breadcrumbs.

PIZZAS

Pizzas are part of growing up, and I've never known a kid not to like them. So here's a home-made variety!

For the dough
½ oz (12 g) dried yeast, or 1 oz (25 g) fresh yeast
warm water
1½ oz (40 g) sunflower margarine
6 oz (175 g) plain flour, sifted
pinch of salt
1 egg
sunflower oil for deep-frying

For the topping
tomatoes, skinned and chopped
olive oil
soft cheese (such as Mozzarella or Bel Paese), sliced

Dissolve the yeast in a very little warm water. Rub the sunflower margarine into the flour and add the salt. Make a well in the centre and put in the egg and the yeast liquid, mix well, then knead to a smooth dough. Put in a floured bowl, cover with a cloth and leave to rise for 2 hours.

Knock back the risen dough and form into lots of little rounds. Allow to rise a second time for about 20 minutes, in a warm spot. Deep-fry in hot oil until golden and puffed, then drain well on kitchen paper. Meanwhile, cook the chopped tomato in a little olive oil.

Put some tomato in the middle of each pizza and top with slices of soft cheese. Place under a hot grill until the cheese melts.

Roger's Chicken B C

A marvellous way of cooking because the rice absorbs all the juices from the chicken and mushrooms as it cooks itself.

4 chicken joints
plain flour
salt and pepper
sunflower oil
8 oz (225 g) rice
½ onion, grated
4 oz (100 g) mushrooms, sliced
sunflower margarine
1 pint (600 ml) chicken stock

Preheat the oven to 180°C/350°F/gas mark 4. Dust the chicken with seasoned flour and brown in a little oil. Meanwhile put the rice and some salt and pepper in a greased casserole, and sprinkle in the grated onion. Sauté the mushrooms in 2 oz (50 g) sunflower margarine and add, with their cooking juices, to the casserole. Arrange the chicken over the top, pour in the stock and dot with a little sunflower margarine. Cover with foil and bake for 1 hour.

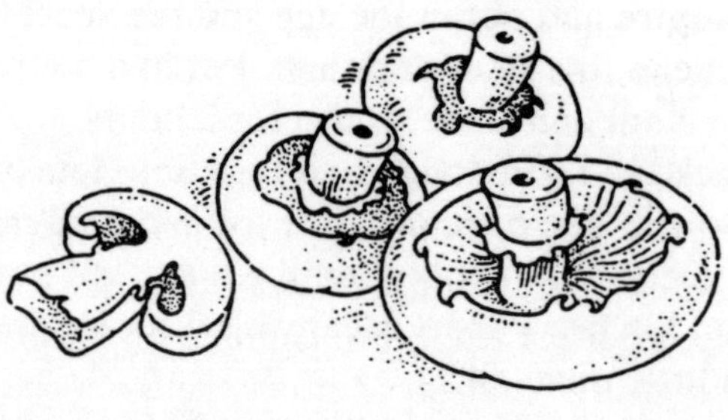

CHICKEN KEBABS

Lovely food for summer days: light chicken kebabs which you can serve with rice, salad and your favourite sauces (see pages 148–152). Beurre Noisette is particularly good.

chicken breasts
mushrooms
salt and pepper
olive oil

Cut the chicken meat into chunks. Cut some mushrooms into wedges and impale them alternately with the chicken chunks on to kebab sticks. Season well and brush liberally with olive oil. Grill under a hot grill, turning and basting frequently with more oil until the chicken is lightly cooked.

PINEAPPLE CHICKEN

Chicken basted with pineapple juice, and served with chopped fruit, is delicious with lightly steamed summer vegetables and a side salad.

chicken joints
salt and pepper
sunflower margarine
canned pineapple

Preheat the oven to 190°C/375°F/gas mark 5. Season the chicken well, dot it with sunflower margarine and bake for 20–25 minutes, basting often with pineapple juice from the can. Cut the pineapple itself into chunks, fry lightly in sunflower margarine, and serve alongside the chicken.

Chicken Wiggle Flan

This tasty quiche of chicken and leek goes well with steamed broccoli and new potatoes.

Oil Pastry (see page 153)
8 oz (225 g) cooked chicken meat
1 small onion, chopped
sunflower margarine
12 oz (350 g) leeks, sliced and cooked
salt and pepper
2 eggs
7 fl oz (200 ml) milk

Line an 8 inch (20 cm) flan dish with oil pastry and bake blind (see page 153).

Preheat the oven to 190°C/375°F/gas mark 5. Slice the chicken and arrange it over the bottom of the pastry case. Soften the onion in a little sunflower margarine and stir in the leeks. Season and spoon over the chicken. Beat the eggs with the milk, season well and pour over the top. Bake for 35–40 minutes.

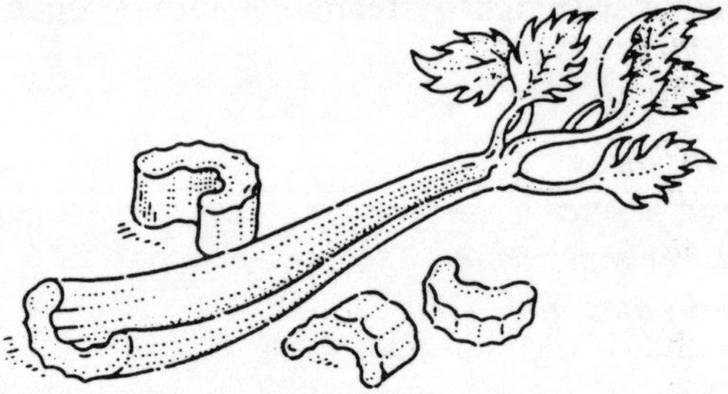

Cheese and Onion Tart

The filling of finely chopped onion turns soft and sweet in the cooking, and mingles with the cheese to make a wonderfully comforting supper dish.

Oil Pastry (see page 153)
1 large onion, chopped finely
6 oz (175 g) cheese, grated
salt and pepper

Line an 8 inch (20 cm) flan dish with oil pastry and bake blind (see page 153).

Preheat the oven to 200°C/400°F/gas mark 6. Fill the centre of the pastry shell with the onion and cover with the grated cheese. Sprinkle with salt and pepper, and bake for 30 minutes.

Sausage Pie

Chipolatas, leeks, tomatoes and cheese contribute their colours to this excellent pie. Serve it with baked potatoes and a vegetable of your choice.

Oil Pastry (see page 153)
8 oz (225 g) chipolata sausages (or vegetarian equivalent)
2 oz (50 g) sunflower margarine
1 onion, chopped
1 lb (450 g) leeks, cooked
4 oz (100 g) cheese, grated
salt and pepper
4 tomatoes, sliced

Line an 8 inch (20 cm) flan dish with oil pastry and bake blind (see page 153).

Preheat the oven to 180°C/350°F/gas mark 4. Fry the chipolatas lightly and cut them in half. Melt the sunflower margarine and sauté the onion. Slice the leeks and add to the onion with half of the cheese, and season. Put into the pastry case and lay the sausages on top, then cover with the sliced tomatoes and sprinkle with the rest of the grated cheese. Bake for 15 minutes.

Barbecue Spare Ribs

Finger food, food to get in a mess with: the kids adore these crisply cooked spare ribs with a sweet-and-sour barbecue sauce. Serve them with crispy noodles (see page 68).

1 lb (450 g) spare ribs of pork
salt

For the sweet and sour sauce
1 tbs tomato purée
4 tbs soy sauce
4 tbs water
1 tbs dark brown sugar
1 tbs vinegar
1 tbs soy sauce
2 tsp mild mustard
salt and pepper

Preheat the oven to 200°C/400°F/gas mark 6. Cut the ribs into individual pieces and season with salt. Roast for 1 hour.

Meanwhile prepare the sauce. Combine all the ingredients in a saucepan and simmer, stirring, for 5 minutes or until well blended. Baste the roasting ribs often with the sauce for the last 20 minutes of the cooking time.

Grated Potato Cake

Grated potatoes make a wonderful dish slowly cooked in a pan until a golden crust forms underneath. Serve this on its own with salad and vegetables, or as a side dish for roast chicken.

1 lb (450 g) potatoes, peeled and grated
2 oz (450 g) sunflower margarine
salt and pepper

Soak the potatoes in cold water, then drain them in a colander and dry thoroughly on a towel. Melt the sunflower margarine in a heavy pan and add the potatoes. Turn until they are covered with the sunflower margarine, and as they begin to soften season them well. Cook, covered, over the lowest possible heat, well pressed down in the pan, for about 45 minutes or until well browned underneath. Turn out on a hot plate and serve.

Funny Fish Ⓒ

A funny mixture perhaps, but it works: fish, rice, lettuce and peas all mixed in a cream sauce and baked until golden. Lovely with a mixed salad.

1 onion, chopped
sunflower margarine
12 oz (350 g) cooked fish, flaked
4 oz (100 g) cooked rice
½ pint (300 ml) Béchamel Sauce (see page 148)
single cream
8 oz (225 g) lettuce, shredded
4 oz (100 g) peas
salt and pepper

Preheat the oven to 190°C/375°F/gas mark 5. Sauté the onion in sunflower margarine over a gentle heat until softened. Mix the fish and rice in a bowl. Add the sautéed onion and béchamel and thin out with cream. Sauté the lettuce briefly in the onion pan in a little more sunflower margarine. Cook the peas until tender and add to the mixture with the lettuce. Season to taste. Pour into an ovenproof dish and bake for 25 minutes.

Stuffed Baked Potatoes

Take large baking potatoes and scrub them well. Allow half a large potato per person, unless they have a gigantic appetite. Pierce with a sharp skewer in two or three places. Bake for 1 hour in a preheated oven at 200°C/400°F/gas mark 6.

Cut the cooked potato in half lengthwise and score the insides with a sharp knife, making a lattice pattern, but leaving the skins intact. Spread with margarine or butter.

Pile your chosen filling on top. Here are some suggestions:

- Mushroom Sauce (see page 149) made with whole button mushrooms
- leeks in cheese sauce
- baked beans
- sweetcorn and spring onion in a little béchamel sauce
- Welsh Rarebit (see page 91)
- chopped walnuts and crumbled blue cheese
- grated Cheddar or Gruyère cheese
- creamed spinach with chopped onion
- ratatouille.

Crispy Noodles

You can obtain rice vermicelli from Chinese grocers, and they make the most sensational crispy noodles in almost no time at all. Serve with any simple dish such as Barbecue Spare Ribs (see page 66), plain grilled fish or roast chicken.

rice vermicelli
hot sunflower or groundnut oil
a little salt

Bring the oil to chip heat, and fry small handfuls of the rice noodles at a time – they puff almost immediately and require the briefest of cooking. Lift out with a slotted spoon and drain on kitchen paper. Keep warm until ready to use.

Desserts and Puddings

There are plenty of recipes to choose from here for rounding off a meal. More than likely a selection will soon be established as firm family favourites. Choose lighter, fruit desserts for summer and warmer weather, and when the greyness of winter is at its dankest you can cheer everyone up with hearty puddings like Roly Poly Pudding and Topsy Turvy Chocolate Pudding. Let the kids help weigh out ingredients, stir, mix and chop – it's a fine way to introduce them to cooking, and give them childhood experiences that they always remember.

Roly Poly Pudding

A delicious roll of light dough encasing fresh fruit of your choice. Try it with pears, apples or plums, and serve with custard or thick yogurt.

1 quantity little Miss Muffin dough *(see page 120)*
1 lb (450 g) peeled and cored (or stoned) fresh fruit, chopped
sugar to taste

Preheat the oven to 200°C/400°F/gas mark 6. Roll out the dough to a long rectangle ¼ inch (5 mm) thick, and sprinkle a little sugar on to it. Cover with the chopped fruit and sprinkle with a little more sugar. Roll up and seal the edges with water. Bake for 30 minutes.

GOOSEBERRY GRUNT

When gooseberries come into season I make the most of them: crumbles, pies, jams – and this delightful pudding which disappears in no time at all. When not in season use thawed, frozen or canned gooseberries, and don't add any water.

1 lb (450 g) gooseberries
4 oz (100 g) sugar
a little ground allspice
water
½ quantity Little Miss Muffin dough (see page 120)

Preheat the oven to 190°C/375°F/gas mark 5. Wash, top and tail the gooseberries. Mix the sugar with the allspice and roll the fruit in the mixture. Put into a greased baking dish with a little water. Roll out the dough and cover the top of the dish. Bake for 30 minutes, until golden, and serve with thick yogurt.

CURRANT TART

A delightful open currant tart which never fails and can be made with storecupboard ingredients. Serve warm or cold with Greek yogurt or single cream.

Sweet Pastry (see page 154)
2 eggs
2 oz (50 g) sugar
1 oz (25 g) plain flour
6 oz (175 g) currants

Line an 8 inch (20 cm) flan dish with the pastry and bake blind (see page 153).

Preheat the oven to 180°C/350°F/gas mark 4. Beat the eggs with the sugar until pale and creamy, then beat in the flour and then mix in the currants. Pour into the pastry case and bake for 40 minutes or until set.

Baked Toffee Apples

Always a winner with the kids, these are a great treat for winter nights, especially Halloween or Bonfire Night. Watch out for sticky fingers . . .

6 apples, cored
1½ oz (40 g) sunflower margarine
2 tbs plain flour
6 oz (175 g) brown sugar
1 tsp vanilla essence

Preheat the oven to 220°C/425°F/gas mark 7. Peel the apples to halfway down. Put them peeled side up into an ovenproof dish.

Melt the sunflower margarine and stir in the flour. Mix well and add the brown sugar and vanilla essence. Spread over the apples. Bake for 20–25 minutes or until the apples are soft.

Pears with Chocolate Sauce [B] [C]

Simplicity itself, for those times when energy is at a low ebb. . . .

Peel some pears and cut into quarters. Remove the stalk and core. Place in a baking dish with a little water and bake at 180°C/350°F/gas mark 4 for 10–12 minutes until tender. Cool, and serve with Chocolate Sauce (see page 87).

Apple Cornflake Crumble

A variation on crumble, this topping is made with cornflakes instead of flour, and makes a crisp, crunchy contrast to the cooked apples underneath. Use bakers or dessert apples. The latter won't need sweetening. Other suitable fruit includes gooseberries, rhubarb and canned apricots.

2 lb (900 g) apples, cored, peeled and sliced
sugar to taste
¼ pint (150 ml) water
8 oz (225 g) cornflakes
4 oz (100 g) sunflower margarine, melted
6 oz (175 g) sugar
pinch each of salt and cinnamon

Preheat the oven to 180°C/350°F/gas mark 4. Arrange the apple slices in a greased ovenproof dish and pour the water over them. Mix the cornflakes with the sunflower margarine, sugar, salt and cinnamon and spread over the apples. Bake for 30 minutes or until the crust is golden.

Paddington's Pie

A biscuit crust case is filled with a light marmalade-flavoured filling. Paddington Bear would love it!

Biscuit Crust (see page 155)
4 oz (100 g) sunflower margarine
4 oz (100 g) icing sugar
3 eggs
2 tbs marmalade (see pages 137–8)

Preheat the oven to 170°C/325°F/gas mark 3. Line a 8 inch (20 cm) greased flan dish with the biscuit crust. Cream the sunflower margarine with the sugar until light. Beat in the eggs and the marmalade and pour into the pastry case. Bake for 1 hour. Serve warm or cold.

Lovely Lemon Pudding

This is gorgeous: the top is cake-like and spongy, and concealed underneath is a lovely lemony liquid.

6 oz (175 g) sugar
4 oz (100 g) plain flour
¼ tsp salt
½ tsp baking powder
3 eggs, separated
4 tbs sugar
rind and juice of 2 lemons
1 oz (25 g) sunflower margarine, melted
¾ pint (450 ml) milk

Preheat the oven to 180°C/350°F/gas mark 4. Sift together the sugar, flour, salt and baking powder. Beat the egg whites until stiff, then beat in the sugar, a spoonful at a time. Beat the egg yolks and add the lemon rind and juice, the melted sunflower margarine and the milk. Stir into the flour mixture and beat until smooth. Fold in the egg whites and pour into a large, greased ovenproof dish. Set in a pan of hot water and bake for 45 minutes. Chill for at least one hour before serving.

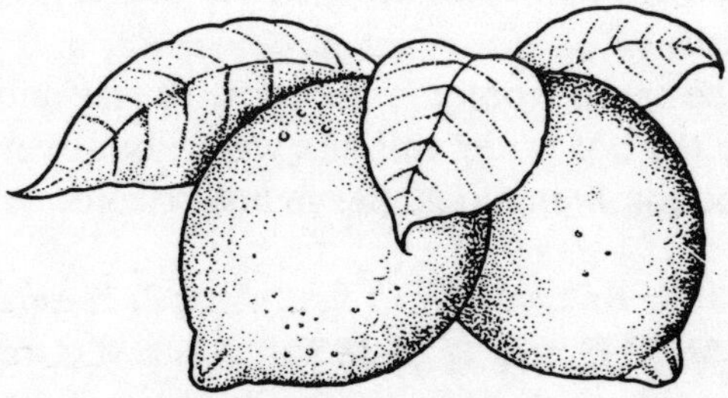

Topsy Turvy Chocolate Pudding

So-called because the sauce which you pour over the sponge mixture before cooking sinks to the bottom, and the cake rises to the top. This has never failed to delight.

3 oz (75 g) self-raising flour
2 tbs cocoa powder
pinch of salt
4 oz (100 g) sunflower margarine
4 oz (100 g) caster sugar
2 eggs
vanilla essence
2 tbs milk

For the sauce
4 oz (100 g) soft brown sugar
2 tbs cocoa powder
½ pint (300 ml) hot water

Preheat the oven to 190°C/375°F/gas mark 5. Sift together the flour, cocoa and salt. In a separate bowl, cream the sunflower margarine and the sugar until light. Mix in the eggs and the vanilla essence and beat to a cream. Add a little of the sifted flour mixture, then gradually fold in the rest with enough milk to make a medium-soft consistency. Pour into a greased ovenproof dish.

To make the sauce, combine the brown sugar and the cocoa. Stir in the hot water and mix well. Pour over the cake mixture. Bake for 40 minutes. Serve hot or cold.

Golden Pear Tart

This fresh pear tart is based on a traditional French recipe, and takes some beating. Serve hot or cold.

Sweet Pastry (see page 154)
2 large pears, peeled and sliced
1 egg and 1 egg yolk
1½ oz (40 g) sugar
1 tbs cornflour
¼ pint (150 ml) single cream
2 tsp vanilla essence

Line a 8 inch (20 cm) flan case with sweet pastry and bake blind (see page 153), then leave to cool.

Preheat the oven to 190°C/375°F/gas mark 5. Arrange the pears in the cooled pastry case. Beat the egg and egg yolk, sugar, cornflour, cream and vanilla and pour over the fruit. Bake for 25 minutes or until puffed and golden.

Peach Crunch

An irresistible topping, light and crunchy and rather like flapjack, is used to cover canned peaches.

1 lb (450 g) canned peaches, drained

For the topping
8 oz (225 g) medium oatmeal
4 oz (100 g) brown sugar
7 fl oz (200 ml) vegetable oil
1 egg, beaten
pinch of salt

Mix the oatmeal, sugar and oil and leave to stand for an hour or two.

Preheat the oven to 180°C/350°F/gas mark 4. Mix the egg and salt into the oatmeal and put into a large, square, greased baking tin. Bake for 30–40 minutes until crisp. Allow to cool.

Crumble the topping. Put the fruit in an ovenproof dish and sprinkle the crumbled topping over it. Bake for 20 minutes.

Apple and Apricot Crunch B C

When improvisation was the name of the game one evening, I came up with this very simple idea of layering apricot jam with apples and topping with biscuit crumbs. We all loved it so much that I've used the formula frequently.

In a greased ovenproof dish make layers of apricot jam and peeled sliced apple rings (sprinkle them with sugar as you go along if the apples are very sour). Top with a thick layer of biscuit crumbs. Dot with sunflower margarine and bake at 180°C/350°F/gas mark 4 for 30 minutes.

Apricot Charlie

A wonderful dessert for a summer's evening: fresh apricots are chopped and folded into thick yogurt or a mixture of yogurt and cream, and sprinkled with Peanut Brittle. As a variation you could use greengages instead of apricots.

1 lb (450 g) ripe apricots, stoned and chopped
½ pint (300 ml) thick Greek yogurt or a mixture of Greek yogurt and whipped double cream
4 oz (100 g) Peanut Brittle (see page 136)

Fold the chopped apricots into the yogurt or whipped cream. Chill. Crush the peanut brittle with a rolling pin and sprinkle over the top.

Fruit Stirabout C

This is a light fruit 'clafoutis', or batter pudding. You can make it with any fruit in season, but here is one of my summer versions. Fresh pitted cherries is another favourite.

4 oz (100 g) plain flour
pinch of salt
2 eggs, separated
½ pint (300 ml) milk
1 oz (25 g) sugar
12 oz (350 g) strawberries or raspberries
1 oz (25 g) sunflower margarine

Preheat the oven to 190°C/375°F/gas mark 5. Sift the flour and the salt into a bowl and make a well in the centre. Put the egg yolks into the well and draw in the flour, mixing to a thick paste. Stir in the milk gradually to make a smooth batter, beating until all the milk is used up. Stir in the sugar and add the fruit.

Heat the margarine in a shallow ovenproof dish until it sizzles. Whisk the egg whites until they are stiff, fold them into the batter, then pour the mixture into the prepared dish. Bake for 30 minutes until risen and browned.

Lovely Layers

Simple to make using any fresh fruit to hand. The middle layers of breadcrumbs stay soft while the top layer dries to make a delicious crunchy topping.

8 oz (225 g) fresh breadcrumbs
2 oz (50 g) sunflower margarine, melted
1½ lb (750 g) mixed fresh fruit (bananas, plums, pears, grapes, etc., peeled and seeded or stoned)
sugar, nutmeg and lemon juice to taste

Preheat the oven to 180°C/350°F/gas mark 4. Mix the breadcrumbs with the melted margarine and cover the bottom of a large ovenproof dish with some of the mixture. Cover the crumbs with a layer of the sliced fruit and sprinkle with sugar, nutmeg and lemon juice. Repeat the layers, ending with the last of the crumbs. Bake for 40 minutes. Serve warm or cold.

LEMON CRUMB PIE

A basic lemon curd tart, this has become a firm favourite over the years . . . and I love it because it is so easily made!

Biscuit Crust (see page 155)
2 eggs, separated
grated juice and rind of 1 lemon
7 oz (200 g) can condensed milk
pinch of salt

Preheat the oven to 170°C/325°F/gas mark 3. Line an 8 inch (20 cm) flan dish with biscuit crust. Beat the egg yolks until thick, then stir in the grated rind and juice of the lemon and the condensed milk and salt. Beat the egg whites until stiff, then fold them into the lemon mixture. Pour into the biscuit shell and bake for 40 minutes. Serve cold.

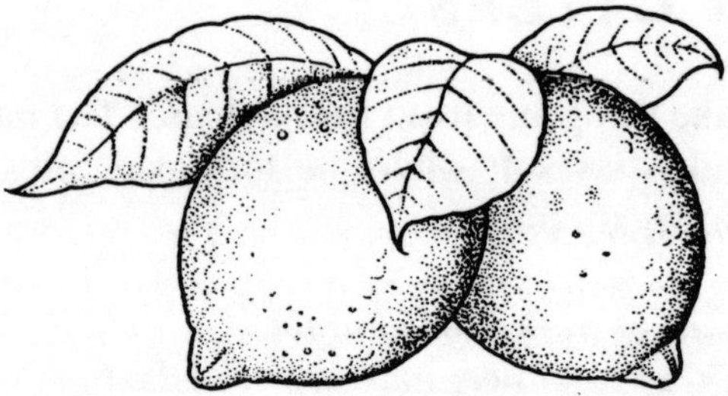

POLAR BEAR PUD [B] [C]

For a special occasion! This is an exotic variety of 'baked Alaska' made with the addition of marshmallows. The secret is to have a very hot oven that will cook the meringue on the outside before the ice cream in the middle has a chance to melt. Kids think it's pure magic!

1½ lb (750 g) mixed fresh fruit, chopped
4 oz (100 g) marshmallows
4 tsp lemon juice
2 egg whites
salt
1 oz (25 g) caster sugar
1 lb (450 g) vanilla ice cream

Preheat the oven to 230°C/450°F/gas mark 8. Put the prepared fruit in the bottom of a greased baking dish. Melt the marshmallows with the lemon juice over a pan of hot water, and leave to cool. Beat the egg whites with the salt until stiff, then beat in the sugar until very firm. Fold in the marshmallow mixture. Cover the fruit with slices of ice cream, then with the meringue mixture, and bake for 5 minutes or until the meringue has browned lightly.

Swiss Roll in the Snow B C

Children love Swiss roll and this is a very simple way of turning it into a fun pudding.

½ Swiss roll
2 eggs, separated
4 oz (100 g) caster sugar
½ pint (300 ml) milk
grated lemon rind

Preheat the oven to 180°C/350°F/gas mark 4. Slice the Swiss roll and put into a well-greased flan dish. Beat the egg yolks with 2 oz (50 g) of the sugar, then add the milk and lemon rind. Pour over the sliced roll, and bake for 15–20 minutes until set. Cool a little.

Beat the egg whites stiffly and add the rest of the sugar, beating until very stiff. Pile on top of the pudding and return to the oven for about 10 minutes to brown.

JOLLY JELLY B C

This jelly, made with satsumas and fresh orange juice, is a welcome change from commercial varieties. Sliced bananas or chopped dessert apple can be used instead of satsumas. For a real party favourite serve with Easy Vanilla Ice Cream (see page 85).

6 satsumas
1 sachet gelatine
1½ pints (900 ml) orange juice

Peel the satsumas and divide them into segments. Melt the gelatine in a little of the orange juice over a low heat until it dissolves, then add to the rest of the juice. Arrange the fruit decoratively in a glass dish and pour the juice carefully over it. Leave in a cool place to set.

☆ *B*anana *B*onanza ☆

It seems that all children love bananas. They are not only ideal for lunch boxes and picnics – they come ready wrapped – but make great sandwich fillings when mashed with a little honey and low-fat cream cheese or dates. There are also hundreds of simple puddings to make with bananas. Try them simply peeled, sliced thinly and sprinkled with lemon juice – or fresh orange juice – and brown sugar, then dotted with butter and baked. Or marinate the slices in fresh lemon juice and sugar, sauté them in butter, roll them up inside thin dessert Pancakes (see page 152) and serve hot, sprinkled with sugar. And what could be easier than bananas and ice cream, with or without Chocolate Sauce (see page 87)?

For other banana recipes see pages 86, 116 and 133.

BANANA AND ALMOND CRUNCH

Bananas baked with a mixture of macaroon, almond and biscuit crumbs. This recipe is as sublime as it is simple.

6 bananas
juice of ½ lemon
sunflower margarine
4 oz (100 g) macaroon crumbs
2 oz (50 g) almond flakes
4 oz (100 g) biscuit crumbs

Preheat the oven to 180°C/350°F/gas mark 4. Cut the bananas in half lengthwise and brush them with lemon juice. Fry them lightly in the sunflower margarine. Arrange them on a greased ovenproof dish and sprinkle with the macaroons, almonds and biscuit crumbs. Dot with more sunflower margarine and bake until golden, about 15 minutes.

BANANA FROST AND FIRE [B] [C]

A kind of 'baked Alaska' with bananas.

2 egg whites
2 oz (50 g) caster sugar
4 bananas
18 fl oz (500 ml) vanilla ice cream

Preheat the oven to 230°C/450°F/gas mark 8. Beat the egg whites until stiff. Beat in the sugar until the mixture is very thick.

Peel the bananas and halve them lengthwise, then cut each piece into three. Arrange half of the banana pieces on the bottom of a greased baking dish and cover with the ice cream. Place the rest of the bananas on top. Spread the stiffly beaten egg whites all over the bananas and ice cream, making sure there are no gaps. Bake for 4–5 minutes. Serve immediately.

Banana and Orange Meringue

Instead of lemon meringue pie, try this banana-based variation along the same lines. The bananas serve as the filling and the base so you don't need a pastry case.

2 oz (50 g) brown sugar
4 bananas
grated rind and juice of 1 orange
juice of ½ lemon
2 egg whites
2 oz (50 g) caster sugar

Preheat the oven to 170°C/325°F/gas mark 3. Sprinkle half of the brown sugar in the bottom of a greased ovenproof dish. Slice the bananas lengthwise and lay on top. Sprinkle with the orange rind, orange and lemon juices and remaining sugar.

Beat the egg whites stiffly, then add the caster sugar. Continue beating until very thick. Spread on top of the bananas and bake for 25 minutes. Serve hot or cold.

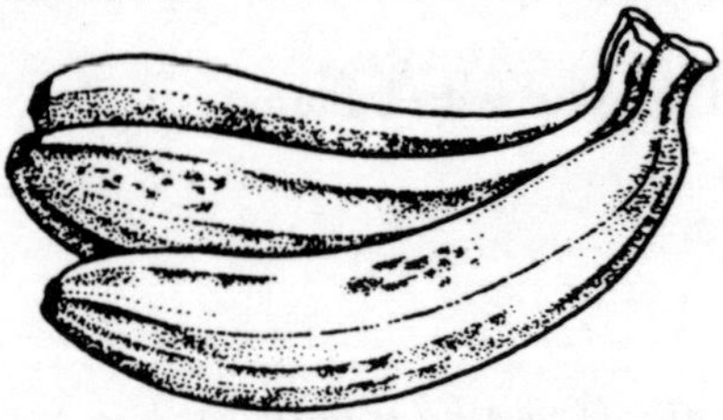

Banana Crumble B C

Bananas seem to have an affinity with walnuts and honey. Here they are baked together with a slightly spicy, oaty crumble topping that can be used with all kinds of fruits.

3 bananas
2 oz (50 g) walnuts
2 tbs clear honey

For the crumble topping
2 oz (50 g) plain flour
1 tsp mixed spice
2 oz (50 g) sunflower margarine
2 tbs caster sugar
2 tbs medium oatmeal

Preheat the oven to 190°C/375°F/gas mark 5. Peel and slice the bananas. Chop the nuts coarsely, combine with the bananas, and pour the mixture into a greased baking dish. Spoon the honey over the top.

To make the topping, sift the flour with the spice, then rub in the sunflower margarine. Add the sugar and oatmeal and mix in lightly. Sprinkle over the banana mixture and bake for 30 minutes.

BANANA NUTKIN Ⓒ

This is a kind of bread-and-butter pudding made with bananas and is wonderfully filling food – excellent fuel for the hungry!

4 slices bread
4 oz (100 g) nuts, chopped
4 bananas, sliced
2 oz (50 g) sugar
2 tsp grated lemon rind
2 eggs
¾ pint (450 ml) milk
nutmeg

Preheat the oven to 180°C/350°F/gas mark 4. Cut the crusts off the bread. Grease a shallow flan tin and place two of the slices of bread on the bottom. Sprinkle with half the nuts, cover with the sliced bananas, then sprinkle with 1 oz (25 g) sugar and the lemon rind. Cover with the remaining nuts and smooth down the top. Finish with the last two slices of bread.

Beat the eggs with the rest of the sugar. Mix in the milk and pour over the bread. Grate a little nutmeg over the top. Bake for 45 minutes. Serve hot.

Banana Fool

A lovely banana fool, flavoured lightly with lemon juice, is topped with chopped peanuts. Serve it with the Sugar Crisps on page 126.

4 bananas
2 oz (50 g) sugar
juice of 1 lemon
½ pint (300 ml) double cream, whipped, or thick yogurt
chopped peanuts

Peel the bananas. Mash them and add the sugar and lemon juice. Heat to boiling point, then press through a sieve, and chill. Fold in the whipped cream and spoon into glasses. Serve chilled, sprinkled with chopped peanuts.

Humpty Dumplings

A roll of light dough encasing a baked banana is one of Life's Good Things. Allow half a banana per person and one quantity of Little Miss Muffin Dough for every four bananas. Serve with thick yogurt or cream.

bananas
lemon juice
sugar
Little Miss Muffin dough (see page 120)
milk

Preheat the oven to 200°C/400°F/gas mark 6. Peel the bananas, slice them lengthwise and cut the slices in half. Marinate them in lemon juice and sugar until softened or for up to half an hour. Roll each one in a little parcel of thinly rolled-out dough. Brush with milk and sprinkle with sugar. Bake for 10 minutes or until golden-brown.

☆ Ice Cream Dreams ☆

Treat-time, and not just for the children – there is the pleasure for you of giving them things they really love! These ice creams with their toppings and sauces are ever-popular and useful at all times of the year, so a supply of ice cream in the freezer will stand you in good stead. And some of the ice creams use cream, others use yogurt, so it's not ALL sin!

Easy Vanilla Ice Cream

This recipe has been my much-repeated standby over the years, and makes the best ice cream I know, with its genuine flavour and light texture. What's more it doesn't require beating during freezing like some home-made ice creams.

¼ pint (150 ml) double cream
1½ oz (40 g) icing sugar, sifted
2 tsp vanilla essence
2 egg whites

Whip the cream with the sifted sugar until it is thick, then flavour with vanilla. Beat the egg whites until very stiff and fold into the cream. Put into a container, cover and freeze.

Two variations that are very good: add chopped, salted peanuts or crushed biscuit crumbs to the cream before folding in the egg whites.

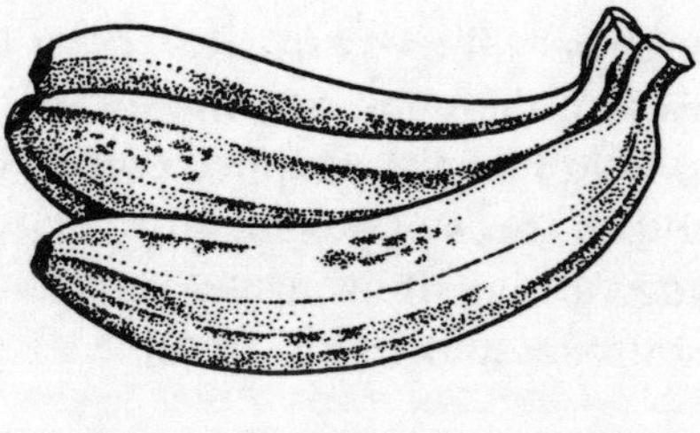

Banana Ice Cream B C

Very easy to make, this ice cream uses evaporated milk instead of cream. Transfer the ice cream from freezer to fridge about 15 minutes before serving to allow to soften a little.

¾ pint (450 ml) evaporated milk
2 eggs, separated
4 oz (100 g) sugar
2 bananas, mashed
juice of 1 lemon
1 tsp vanilla essence
pinch of salt

Beat the evaporated milk until thick. Beat the egg yolks with the sugar until thick, then beat in the milk. Stir in the bananas, lemon juice and vanilla.

Beat the egg whites with the salt until they are stiff. Fold into the banana mixture. Freeze. Stir the semi-frozen mixture after about 2–3 hours, to break up any ice crystals. Return to the freezer.

Peach Ice Cream

A simple version of ice cream which you can make using either cream or Greek yogurt. A great standby to have in the freezer.

½ pint (300 ml) double cream or thick Greek yogurt
1 lb (450 g) can peaches in natural juice

Whip the cream or beat the yogurt. Reserve a few pieces of peach for decoration, then liquidise the rest with half of the juice in the can. Fold into the whipped cream. Freeze, and serve decorated with slices of peach.

This is a wonderful way of using any canned or fresh fruit. Mangoes, for example, make a memorable ice cream.

YOGURT ICE CREAM Ⓒ

Into some plain yogurt fold honey to taste and some chopped nuts and raisins. Cover and freeze. Yogurt ice cream is also lovely with a little caster sugar added to it before freezing.

CHOCOLATE SAUCE

Dark, thick and oh-so divine on vanilla ice cream. Add a slice of banana for a traditional banana split. Liquidised canned peaches are also excellent on ice cream.

½ pint (300 ml) boiling water
8 oz (225 g) sugar
pinch of salt
2 oz (50 g) cocoa
1 tsp vanilla essence

Mix together all the ingredients except the vanilla essence and stir over a moderate heat until smooth. Cook for 10 minutes, then flavour with the vanilla. Store in an airtight jar in the fridge.

BUTTERSCOTCH SAUCE

A scrumptious dark syrup to pour over vanilla ice cream – a treat at any time of the year.

4 oz (100 g) dark brown sugar
¼ pint (150 ml) golden syrup
½ tsp salt
1 oz (25 g) sunflower margarine
1 tsp vanilla essence

Heat the sugar with the syrup and simmer for 10 minutes. Add the rest of the ingredients and stir well.

Ice Cream Topping

Gilding the lily, you might say, but crumbling this topping over ice cream has proved a great treat for my kids!

1 oz (25 g) sunflower margarine
2 oz (50 g) soft brown sugar
2 oz (50 g) crushed cornflakes

Melt the sunflower margarine with the sugar, and when it has dissolved add the cornflakes. When cold, crumble over ice cream.

Knickerbocker Glory

The classic ice cream treat, part of the mythology of childhood – this is a party piece.

3 different colour jellies
ice cream
sliced bananas, grapes, raspberries, etc.
whipped cream

Place tablespoons of the jellies alternately with the ice cream in a glass, then alternate layers of fruit and ice cream to the top of the glass. Finish with a swirl of whipped cream.

Cheerful Cherry Bomb

Another good pudding to serve at children's parties.

Break some Meringues (see page 124) into small pieces and use to cover the bottom of a serving dish. Cover with scoops of Easy Vanilla Ice Cream (see page 85), and decorate with whipped cream and halved glacé cherries (or fresh black cherries in season!) Serve at once.

As a variation, heat some canned black cherries in the juices from the can and pour them over the top of each serving.

Ice Cream Cake

What could be simpler than this? Again, it makes an impressive party pudding.

Put a thin layer of Swiss roll or any sponge cake in the bottom of a serving dish, and make two more layers alternating Easy Vanilla Ice Cream (see page 85). Decorate with whipped cream and sprinkle with chopped glacé cherries and nuts. Serve immediately.

Icebergs

For nut-freaks, this is your number!

Put scoops of ice cream into glasses and cover with chopped nuts – a mixture of walnuts, hazelnuts and almonds is best if you have them all. Garnish your iceberg with a sprig of mint.

Chopped nuts are always scrumptious on ice cream: try chopped peanuts on chocolate ice cream.

Flowerpots

In the summer when the garden is full of flowers, fill some decorated pots or bowls with ice cream, smooth down the top and cover with grated chocolate. Pick some flowers, wrap the stems in foil so that they are sealed, and set them in little bunches in the pots. They look as if they are growing out of the earth.

Snack Meals

There are so many occasions when you have to cook on the run – demands are being made on you from all directions, people are in a hurry, they are coming in and out at different times and nothing can be scheduled. Don't despair: this section is for you! These ideas are for tasty and nutritious snack meals which can be quickly and easily prepared. Things on toast, such as baked beans, poached eggs or grilled mushrooms, make the speediest of snacks and I've included plenty more ideas for toast-based snacks. Cheese and ham are useful standbys so don't be surprised to find them cropping up again and again in this section. Children love them.

Salami Scrambles

A mouthwatering scramble of salami, celery, eggs and a little cheese is heaped on to crisp, baked bread.

slices of bread
sunflower margarine, melted
slices of salami cut into strips
celery, finely chopped
eggs
a little grated cheese
salt and pepper

Preheat the oven to 200°C/400°F/gas mark 6. Cut off the crusts from the bread, then brush the slices with melted sunflower margarine. Bake for 10–12 minutes. Meanwhile sauté the salami and celery in margarine, then scramble some eggs with them. Add grated cheese, season well and serve on the bread.

OMELETTES C

Omelettes are one obvious answer to a quick snack meal. There are endless variations on the theme, but here is one with a difference. It can be served hot or cold.

½ pint (300 ml) milk
2 oz (50 g) fresh wholemeal breadcrumbs
6 eggs, well beaten
salt and pepper
1 oz (25 g) sunflower margarine
2 oz (50 g) diced cooked chicken or ham

Warm the milk, then soak the breadcrumbs in it. Add the well beaten eggs. Season to taste. Melt the margarine in a frying pan and when it is sizzling pour in the egg mixture. When the bottom begins to set, scatter on the diced chicken or ham. Fold the omelette over and cut into portions.

WELSH RAREBIT B C

This is an old favourite with children and adults alike.

Per person
2 eggs
1 tbs milk
about 1 oz (25 g) grated Cheddar or Edam cheese
salt and pepper
1 slice wholemeal toast

Beat the eggs, then mix in the milk and grated cheese. Season, heap on to toast, and put under a hot grill until lightly set.

Speedy Sardines

Four ideas for ringing the changes with a can of sardines:

- Halve some sardines carefully, dip in seasoned flour, beaten egg and breadcrumbs and fry them in hot oil until crisp and golden. Serve piping hot.
- Make a Welsh Rarebit (see page 91) and pour it over sardines on toast. Grill until lightly puffed and golden.
- Lay slices of cheese over some sardines on a flat, greased ovenproof dish and grill until the cheese bubbles.
- Mash sardines with softened sunflower margarine and lemon juice, season with pepper, and put on to squares of fried bread. Heat through and serve.

Stuffed Tunny Buns

A deliciously soft-textured filling of tuna, cheese and hard-boiled eggs inside a soft bap is heated through in the oven: a brilliant snack meal. Canned salmon can also be used.

Makes 6

1 oz (25 g) grated cheese
2 hard-boiled eggs, chopped
1 small can tuna
5 tbs mayonnaise
some chopped onion and pickle
6 soft baps

Preheat the oven to 180°C/350°F/gas mark 4. Mix the first five ingredients together, and stuff into the soft baps. Wrap in foil and bake for 30 minutes.

Quick Fish Gratin

This quick gratin of fish and cauliflower has the addition of cracker crumbs to make it substantial, warming food.

12 oz (350 g) white fish, cooked and flaked
1 egg, beaten
1 onion, chopped finely
1 cauliflower, cooked and separated into florets
4 oz (100 g) savoury cracker crumbs
¼ pint (150 ml) milk
salt and pepper
2 oz (50 g) Cheddar cheese, grated

Preheat the oven to 170°C/325°F/gas mark 3. Combine the fish, beaten egg and onion, and mix well. Add the cauliflower, cracker crumbs and milk. Season and mix well. Put into a greased ovenproof dish and top with the grated cheese. Bake for 30 minutes.

Ham Patties

These little patties are quick and easy to make, and very tasty. Serve hot with your kids' favourite salad and some buttered noodles or a baked potato.

Makes 10

8 oz (225 g) ham, minced
2 eggs, beaten
2 oz (50 g) dried breadcrumbs
soy sauce
salt and pepper
milk or water
sunflower oil

Mix together the ham, eggs and breadcrumbs and season to taste with soy sauce, salt and pepper. Add enough milk or water to shape into patties. Fry in oil until golden on both sides.

Crusty Ham

A fabulous variation on the hot sandwich. Crisp ham sandwiches are topped with a ball of cheese paste and baked until it melts.

thin slices of bread
sunflower margarine
slices of ham
grated cheese
salt and pepper

Preheat the oven to 200°C/400°F/gas mark 6. Cut the crusts off the bread, then dip the slices into some melted sunflower margarine. Cut the slices of ham to the same size and make sandwiches. Cut into quarters.

Work to a paste some grated cheese, sunflower margarine, salt and pepper and shape into small balls. Put one on each sandwich quarter and bake for 10 minutes.

Cheese Dogs

Cut a long slit in each frankfurter (or vegetarian substitute) and tuck into it a long thin slice of cheese. Grill, cheese side up, until the cheese melts. Serve inside a long wholemeal roll.

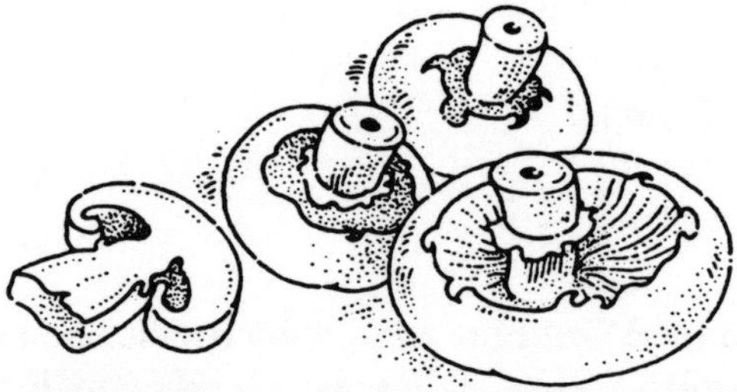

SAUSAGE SNACKS

- Fry rounds of sausagemeat (or vegetarian substitute) in a little sunflower oil until crisp. Add some more oil to the pan and fry rings of cored, sliced apple until golden on both sides. Serve hot. This is also good with pineapple rings instead of the apple.
- Shape well-seasoned sausagemeat (or vegetarian substitute) into croquettes and dip in beaten egg and then breadcrumbs. Fry in hot, shallow vegetable oil until browned all over.
- Wrap rolls of sausagemeat (or vegetarian substitute) in Little Miss Muffin dough (see page 119) and bake at 200°C/400°F/gas mark 6 for 25 minutes.

SAUSAGE BURGERS

An excellent, tasty variation on the theme of the burger. You can make the burgers with minced meat instead of sausagemeat, if you prefer.

Makes 8

1 onion, chopped
2 tbs sunflower oil
1 lb (450 g) sausagemeat (or vegetarian substitute)
2–3 tbs fresh breadcrumbs
salt and pepper
1 egg, beaten
flour
bread rolls, warmed

Fry the onion in the oil until soft. Mix with the sausagemeat and breadcrumbs, season and bind with the egg. Shape into eight patties, roll in flour and fry on both sides until golden. Serve inside the warm rolls.

Hickety Pickety Chicken [B] [C]

Layers of chicken and cooked spinach topped with béchamel sauce, and baked until golden, makes wonderful food from leftovers.

Put leftover cooked chicken meat, cut into strips, on a bed of spinach or broccoli which has been cooked and drained. Cover with a little more spinach or broccoli and top with Béchamel Sauce (see page 148) and a light sprinkling of grated cheese or fresh breadcrumbs. Dot with sunflower margarine and bake at 200°C/400°F/gas mark 6 for 15 minutes.

Shepherd's Secret

A scrumptious version of shepherd's pie, topped with crushed potato crisps for a change.

1 onion, grated
1 lb (450 g) lean mince (or vegetarian substitute)
a little sunflower oil
salt and pepper
8 oz (225 g) cooked leftover vegetables such as carrots, leeks, broad beans, green beans etc
3–4 tbs Béchamel Sauce (see page 148)
1–2 large packets potato crisps

Preheat the oven to 200°C/400°F/gas mark 6. Mix the onion with the mince. Fry in oil until browned, season well and add the vegetables with a little béchamel sauce to moisten the mixture. Put into a greased ovenproof dish. Crush the potato crisps, spread them over the top and bake for 10–15 minutes.

HASTY HAGGIS

A fast fry of mince, onion and oatmeal makes a nourishing quick meal for hungry people. Lovely with jacket potatoes.

1 onion, chopped finely
2 tbs sunflower oil
8 oz (225 g) lean mince
8 oz (225 g) bacon rashers, chopped finely
a little water or tomato juice
salt and pepper
2 oz (50 g) medium oatmeal

Fry the onion in the oil. Add the mince and the chopped bacon and brown them. Moisten with a little tomato juice or water, season, and scatter on the oatmeal. Simmer for a few minutes. Serve hot.

MUSHROOM MUNCH [B] [C]

A scrumptious dish: grated potatoes topped with mushrooms in a béchamel sauce, and baked for a long time so that the flavours and textures mingle. Serve with a tossed salad.

4 oz (100 g) mushrooms, sliced
sunflower margarine
¾ pint (450 ml) Béchamel Sauce (see page 148)
1 lb (450 g) potatoes, peeled and grated
salt and pepper

Preheat the oven to 180°C/350°F/gas mark 4. Sauté the mushrooms in a little sunflower margarine. Add to the béchamel sauce and mix well. Put the potatoes into a greased ovenproof dish and season, then pour the mushroom and béchamel mixture over the potatoes. Bake for 1¼ hours.

Mophead Mushrooms

This is a kind of soufflé-omelette on toast, and both looks and tastes wonderful. Serve with some lightly steamed vegetables.

4 oz (100 g) sliced mushrooms
1 tsp grated onion
1½ oz (40 g) sunflower margarine
2 eggs, separated
2 oz (50 g) cheese, grated
salt, pepper and cayenne
4 slices bread
butter

Sauté the mushrooms and onion in the margarine. Combine the egg yolks, cheese and seasonings, then stir in the onion and mushroom mixture. Beat the egg whites stiffly and fold in. Toast the bread on one side only. Butter the other side and heap the mushroom mixture on top. Put under a hot grill until puffed and golden.

Topping Tomatoes

Simple layers of tomatoes, mushrooms, breadcrumbs and cheese are baked to make a mouthwatering supper dish. Serve with a tossed mixed salad.

4 tomatoes, skinned and sliced
2 oz (50 g) mushrooms, sliced
2 oz (50 g) fresh breadcrumbs
2 oz (50 g) Cheddar cheese, grated
salt and pepper
1 oz (25 g) sunflower margarine

Preheat the oven to 180°C/350°F/gas mark 4. Grease a baking dish and put in layers of tomatoes, mushrooms, breadcrumbs and cheese, seasoning each layer with salt and pepper as you go along, and ending with a layer of breadcrumbs. Dot with margarine and bake for 30 minutes.

Crisp Tomatoes

Slice some tomatoes and season them well. Dip the slices into medium oatmeal and fry in sunflower or olive oil until browned and crisp.

Crumby Tomatoes

Layers of thinly sliced tomatoes and fried breadcrumbs are baked until piping hot. Lovely with a tossed salad.

Fry 6 tbs dried breadcrumbs in vegetable oil until golden. Drain on kitchen paper. Sprinkle half of them over the bottom of a greased baking dish. Thinly slice 3 large tomatoes and arrange on top. Season and top with the rest of the crumbs. Bake at 200°C/400°F/gas mark 6 for 15–20 minutes.

Tomato Mounds

Simplicity itself.

Top halved tomatoes with mashed potato, or puréed leftover vegetables, brush with beaten egg and bake at 200°C/400°F/gas mark 6 until golden.

POTATO AND CHEESE PUFFS

This is a kind of potato and cheese soufflé – deliciously comforting food made in a matter of minutes.

4 oz (100 g) Cheddar cheese, grated
¾ pint (450 ml) milk
1½ lb (750 g) mashed potato
1 onion, chopped
salt and pepper
2 eggs, separated

Preheat the oven to 200°C/400°F/gas mark 6. Melt the cheese in the milk over a low heat. Add the mashed potato, onion, seasoning and egg yolks. Beat the egg whites stiffly and fold into the mixture. Bake for 20–25 minutes until browned.

POTATO STICKS

Mix some leftover mashed potatoes with a little melted sunflower margarine. Chill. Pat out to ¾ inch (2 cm) rectangles and cut into strips. Brush with beaten egg. Sprinkle with sesame seeds, pressing them into each side, then place on a baking sheet and bake at 220°C/425°F/gas mark 7 for about 20–25 minutes, until crisp and golden.

POTATO CROQUETTES [B] [C]

For variety you can add chopped onion, grated cheese or minced ham or chicken to the mixture. They can be prepared in advance and chilled until required.

1 lb (450 g) cooked potatoes
1 oz (450 g) sunflower margarine
a little milk
salt and pepper
beaten egg
breadcrumbs
sunflower oil

Mash the potatoes with the sunflower margarine and milk over a gentle heat, and season to taste. Chill. Shape into long rolls, dip in egg and crumbs, and fry in oil until golden.

Grocer's Bake

This is the easiest of standbys, and quite delicious. Instead of canned tomatoes you can use any vegetables to hand – marrow or leeks both work very well. Cook lightly first, then drain and mix with the other ingredients.

4 tbs medium oatmeal
4 oz (100 g) grated cheese
14 oz (400 g) can tomatoes, drained
3–4 tbs milk
salt and pepper

Preheat the oven to 200°C/400°F/gas mark 6. Mix all the ingredients together and season well. Place in an ovenproof dish and bake for 25 minutes.

Cheese Hash [C]

Home-cooking *par excellence*, this is a version of 'hash' or potato cake made with cheese. It turns out a beautiful golden brown.

6 new potatoes
2 oz (50 g) cheese, grated
1 onion, chopped
1 oz (25 g) sunflower margarine
salt and pepper
extra grated cheese

Boil the potatoes in their skins, cool them, then grate them coarsely. Mix with the grated cheese. Gently fry the onion in the sunflower margarine until soft, and add to the potato.

Season with salt and pepper. Press the mixture down well in a greased frying pan and cook over a low heat until a thick brown crust has formed underneath. Sprinkle with more grated cheese and finish under the grill.

FRED'S NOODLES Ⓒ

Noodles are a great standby for easy eats, and the simple idea of serving them tossed in good butter and some grated cheese is unbeatable. Serve with a crisp green salad.

8 oz (225 g) noodles
2 oz (50 g) unsalted butter
grated Cheddar cheese

Cook the noodles, drain, then add the butter and turn until the noodles are well coated. Heap on to a platter and sprinkle with grated cheese. Toss again until the cheese melts, and serve immediately.

VEGETABLE STIRABOUT

An excellent way of using leftover lentils, and leeks or other vegetables, this is made in no time at all yet produces a nourishing snack meal.

2 oz (50 g) cooked green or brown lentils
1 oz (25 g) sunflower margarine
2 leeks, cooked
grated Cheddar cheese

Stir the lentils gently in some of the sunflower margarine over a low heat. Warm the leeks in the remaining sunflower margarine, then stir all together. Sprinkle with a little grated cheese and brown under the grill.

Golden Cheese Balls

Serve these light cheese balls with a green salad and crusty bread.

Makes 16

2 egg whites
pinch of salt
4 oz (100 g) cheese, grated
2 oz (50 g) plain flour, sifted
salt and pepper
dried breadcrumbs or crushed savoury cracker crumbs
sunflower or groundnut oil

Beat the egg whites stiffly with a pinch of salt. Add the cheese and flour and season well. Form into balls, roll in breadcrumbs or cracker crumbs and fry in oil until golden-brown. Serve hot.

Fried Cheese

These mouthwatering morsels make a superlative snack, served with a green salad.

Cut slices of soft cheese (Bel Paese is best) ¼ inch (½ cm) thick. Dip in flour, beaten egg and breadcrumbs and fry in hot vegetable oil. Drain on paper and serve at once.

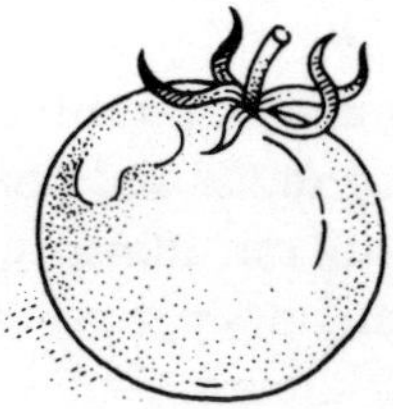

Sweetcorn Fritters

These delectable fritters make an unbeatable snack meal, excellent with a tomato salad and granary bread.

8 oz (225 g) can sweetcorn, drained
1 onion, chopped
4 tbs self-raising flour
4 tbs chutney
4 eggs, beaten lightly
salt and pepper
sunflower oil for deep frying

Mix all the ingredients and season well. Scoop into balls with a small spoon and deep-fry until golden-brown and puffed. Drain on kitchen paper and serve.

Little Cheese Parcels

Little triangles of pastry with melted cheese inside, deep-fried until golden, make a great treat for the kids. They usually eat them as fast as you can make them!

4 oz (100 g) plain flour
pinch of salt
1½ oz (40 g) sunflower margarine
a little soy sauce
1 tbs boiling water
4 oz (100 g) grated Gruyère cheese
ground black pepper
sunflower oil for deep frying

Sift together the flour and salt and rub in the sunflower margarine. Mix in the soy sauce and boiling water to make a stiff dough. Knead and roll out thinly. Cut into 3 inch (7.5 cm) squares. Liberally pepper the grated cheese and place a spoonful on each square. Fold in half to make a triangle and seal the edges with water. Deep-fry until golden. Drain on kitchen paper and eat as soon as possible.

French Fried Sandwiches

Cut the crusts off slices of bread and spread the slices with sunflower margarine mixed with a little mild mustard. Fill with chopped ham, Gruyère or Cheddar cheese, chicken or corned beef. Press them down well and chill.

Dip the sandwiches in beaten egg mixed with a little top of the milk or cream, and fry in sunflower oil until golden brown on both sides. Serve hot.

Hot Peanut Butter Sandwiches

These are scrumptious: the butter permeates the bread and makes it soft, and the outside remains slightly crisp.

Cut some thin slices of bread and remove the crusts. Butter the slices and sandwich them with home-made Peanut Butter (see page 142). Bake in a low oven (150°C/300°F/gas mark 2) for 15 minutes.

As a variation, add a little crisped bacon to the filling. Or add thinly sliced banana to the filling and serve cold.

Pepper and Bacon Toasties

Cut some rounds out of slices of bread with a pastry cutter or small glass. Toast the rounds on one side and butter the other side. Stiffly beat some egg whites and fold in chopped red or green pepper and seasonings. Fold in some crisped bacon, heap on to the buttered side of the bread and grill for about 3–5 minutes, until golden-brown and set.

Bacon and Cheese Toasted Sandwiches

Slice some bread and spread with butter or margarine. Sandwich with crisped bacon and grated cheese. Put under a hot grill until toasted on both sides.

Tunny Fish Toasted Sandwiches

Toast slices of bread, butter them and sandwich thickly with some tuna mashed with finely chopped tomatoes. Warm through rapidly in a moderate oven and serve.

Other Fillings for Toasted Sandwiches:

- Minced ham and mustard.
- Finely chopped, sautéed kidneys and crisped, crumbled bacon.
- Crispy bacon and lettuce.
- Slices of frankfurter and diced pineapple.
- Chunks of fried fish mixed with scrambled eggs.

Goodies on Toast

- Sardines mashed with lemon juice and chopped celery.
- Scrambled egg with anchovy or flaked kipper.
- Apples fried in sunflower margarine and topped with crisped bacon.
- Finely sliced kidneys fried in sunflower margarine with a little mustard.
- Tuna fish mashed with a little mayonnaise, chopped hard-boiled egg and capers.
- Grilled mushrooms or tomatoes.
- Sardine butter, mayonnaise, chopped gherkins and capers.

Lunch Boxes and Picnics

Lunch boxes and picnics require endless variations on the theme of the sandwich. A sandwich can be the best or the worst of meals – at best unbeatable, and a nutritionist's dream. At worst, pre-sliced plastic bread sheltering slices of plastic ham and wilting lettuce hardly merit the same title.

With a little flair and imagination, packed meals can be mouth-watering and satisfying, and are quickly and easily prepared. As a variation on the theme, a ploughman's lunch is a wonderful meal and children enjoy it enormously – and it is one that they can help you to prepare!

ZEBRAS

One fun variation on the sandwich theme, to ring the changes in the daily lunch box, is to use a slice of white bread for the top and brown bread for the bottom.

In the summer, chopped watercress makes a delicious filling, mixed with cream cheese or low-fat soft cheese. Or make your bi-coloured sandwiches with a filling of chopped hard-boiled eggs and shredded lettuce, mixed with a generous quantity of mayonnaise or salad cream.

This filling is perhaps the most scrumptious of all: chunks of smoked mackerel mixed with creamy, lightly scrambled eggs, well seasoned with salt and pepper, cooled, then sandwiched between the layers of buttered bread.

Pinwheels

Cut off the crusts from thin slices of bread. Butter the slices and spread them with your chosen filling. Roll them up, fasten them with cocktail sticks, and chill.

Pancake Sandwiches

Make a mixture of cooked, chopped chicken, fish or mushrooms, a little thick Mild Mustard Sauce (see page 149), and a little cream. Make layers with Pancakes (see page 152) and cut in wedges. Or roll up and pack in cling-film for a picnic or lunch box.

Cock-Eyed Loaf

Picnic food *par excellence*.

Mix a can of sardines with a couple of chopped hard-boiled eggs, some shredded lettuce and Mayonnaise (page 151). Cut the crusts off a sandwich loaf and slice the bread several times lengthwise. Butter the slices and sandwich with the filling. Press under a weight and chill. To serve, cover with mayonnaise and cut in vertical slices. Garnish with chopped gherkin.

Tommy Tucker's Supper Ⓒ

A creamy, summery mixture of lightly scrambled egg cooked with tomatoes and cheese, this makes a sandwich filling with a difference.

2 large tomatoes, fresh or canned
2 oz (50 g) sunflower margarine
4 oz (100 g) Cheddar cheese, grated
1 egg, well beaten
salt and pepper

If using fresh tomatoes, scald and peel them. Chop the tomatoes finely. Melt the sunflower margarine in a frying pan, and add the tomatoes and the cheese. Lastly add the beaten egg and seasonings. Simmer for 2–3 minutes and allow to cool before using as a filling for sandwiches, rolls or a baguette.

Scandinavian Open Sandwiches

Make some light toast, or use crispbread, and spread with mayonnaise on one side. Top it with:

- Crisped bacon, lettuce and tomato.
- Thin steaks cooked rare, or to individual preference, with fried onions.
- Grated cheese and sliced cucumber.
- Chopped chicken and watercress.

Chicken Loaf [B] [C]

A delightfully light loaf which, sliced, is a versatile ingredient of a lunch box or picnic. Eat it as it comes, with a salad, or on a piece of crispbread *à la* open sandwich, or in a salad roll.

8 oz (225 g) cooked chicken meat, chopped
2 oz (50 g) fresh breadcrumbs
½ pint (300 ml) milk
2 eggs
salt and pepper
soy sauce
lemon juice
2 celery sticks, chopped

Preheat the oven to 170°C/325°F/gas mark 3. Mix all the ingredients together and put into a greased 1 lb (450 g) loaf tin. Set in a tin of boiling water and bake for 40 minutes or until a knife inserted in the centre comes out clean. Allow to stand for 15 minutes before turning out. Chill.

HOPPIN' HAM LOAF B C

Creamy in texture and rich in flavour, slices of this ham loaf make marvellous picnic food. Or put them into a roll or baguette for a lunch box.

2 oz (50 g) granary bread, sliced
½ pint (300 ml) milk
1 lb (450 g) cooked ham, minced
chopped parsley
salt, pepper and ground mace
1 egg, beaten

Preheat the oven to 170°C/325°F/gas mark 3. Cut the crusts off the bread. Heat the milk to boiling point, pour it over the slices of bread and mash the mixture until smooth. Add the ham and parsley and mix well. Season and add the beaten egg. Put into a greased 1 lb (450 g) loaf tin and stand in a pan of hot water. Bake for 1 hour. Cool on a rack, and turn out when cold.

SALMON LOAF

An easy-to-make fish loaf that could also be made with tuna or mackerel. Delicious with tomatoes or cucumber and served either in a salad roll or on a picnic plate.

1 lb (450 g) can salmon
4 eggs, beaten
4 oz (100 g) sunflower margarine, melted
3 oz (75 g) fresh breadcrumbs
salt and pepper

Preheat the oven to 180°C/350°F/gas mark 4. Mash the fish, beat in the beaten eggs and melted margarine, then stir in the breadcrumbs. Season to taste. Turn into a greased 2 lb (900 g) loaf tin and bake standing in a pan of hot water, for 1 hour. Cool on a rack, and turn out after 15 minutes or when cold.

Potato Crisps

Home-made crisps are the best of all!

Peel some potatoes and slice them very thinly – as thin as paper. Use the slicer on the side of a cheese grater for quickest results. Dry them on kitchen paper and deep-fry in very hot vegetable oil. Drain on kitchen paper and serve sprinkled with salt. Store in airtight jars.

Crisplets

Tiny grated flakes of potato cooked until crisp and golden: very moreish!

Peel some potatoes and grate them on the coarse side of the grater. Deep-fry in very hot vegetable oil (200°C/400°F) until golden and crisp.

Deep-Fried Rice

A wonderful way of making something special with leftover rice.

Deep-fry some cooked rice until golden-brown and crisp. Lift out carefully with a slotted spoon. Drain on kitchen paper, sprinkle with salt, and serve as a snack.

SUNFLOWER SEEDS

Browned sunflower seeds are a wonderful nibble, and a nutritious addition to the kids' lunch boxes.

Fry sunflower seeds in vegetable oil until browned all over, tossing them as they cook. Drain on kitchen paper, sprinkle with salt and serve when they are cool.

PEANUT STRAWS

A variation of the cheese straw, studded with chopped peanuts. A treat for the kids' lunch boxes.

3 oz (75 g) plain flour
3 oz (75 g) sunflower margarine
3 oz (75 g) Cheddar cheese, grated
salt and pepper
1–1½ oz (25–40 g) dry-roasted peanuts

Preheat the oven to 180°C/350°F/gas mark 4. Sift the flour, rub in the margarine, then add the cheese with the seasonings. Knead to a paste and roll out thinly. Put the nuts in the blender and chop them roughly. Press them into the pastry, then cut into long straws and place on a well-greased baking tray. Bake for 10 minutes, until golden and crisp.

CHEESE BUTTERFLIES

Delicate cheese morsels which grace an 'alfresco' meal with their elegance.

Makes 24

6 oz (175 g) cheese, grated
4 oz (100 g) sunflower margarine
4 oz (100 g) plain flour
¼ tsp salt

Cream the cheese with the margarine, then blend in the flour and salt. Pat into a firm ball and chill for at least 1 hour.

Roll out thinly and cut into butterfly shapes with a cutter (or use any other pretty shaped cutters you may have). Place on a greased baking sheet and chill again.

Preheat the oven to 200°C/400°F/gas mark 6. Bake for 7–10 minutes.

Walnut Bread

A delicious walnut bread which packs perfectly into the lunch box as a change from ordinary bread, and can also be eaten for 'afters'.

Makes 2 loaves

2 eggs
4 oz (100 g) dark brown sugar
1 lb (450 g) plain flour
4 tsp baking powder
½ tsp salt
1 pint (600 ml) milk
6 oz (175 g) walnuts, chopped

Beat the eggs well and stir in the sugar. Sift together in a bowl the flour, baking powder and salt, and add to the egg mixture alternately with the milk. Stir in the nuts. Put into two greased 1 lb (450 g) loaf tins and allow to stand for 30 minutes.

Preheat the oven to 180°C/350°F/gas mark 4. Bake the loaves for 40 minutes until a knife inserted in the centre comes out clean.

Cheese Scones

Great for an informal picnic lunch, these cheese scones are delicious simply lightly buttered, to go with a salady meal. Perfect for the lunch box, too.

Makes 15–18

Add 4 oz (100 g) grated cheese to one quantity of Little Miss Muffin dough (see page 120) before adding the milk. Proceed with the instructions for the muffins, and then cut into triangles. Bake on a greased baking sheet and bake at 230°C/450°F/gas mark 8 for 15 minutes.

Orange Muffins

For a picnic tea in the fields, or as a sweet treat in the lunch box, these orange muffins are light and tasty.

Makes 18

12 oz (350 g) plain flour
2 tsp baking powder
4 tbs sugar
½ tsp salt
1 egg
juice of 2 oranges and rind of 1 orange
4 oz (100 g) sunflower margarine, melted
a little milk

Preheat the oven to 200°C/400°F/gas mark 6. Sift the dry ingredients together in a bowl and make a well in the centre. Beat the egg and add with the orange juice and rind and the melted margarine. Mix quickly to a dough with enough milk to thin out. Drop spoonfuls into greased muffin tins and bake for 20 minutes.

Quaker Crunch

Perfect to pack into the lunch box for the sweet course, these are delectably crisp, satisfying food.

4 oz (100 g) sunflower margarine
4 oz (100 g) brown sugar
6 oz (175 g) porridge oats

Preheat the oven to 190°C/375°F/gas mark 5. Cream together the margarine and the sugar until soft, then stir in the oats until well blended. Spread on a shallow, greased baking sheet, pressing down evenly and bake for 25 minutes. Cut into squares when cool, then turn out when cold.

Peanut Biscuits

Crisp, golden and nutty, these crunchy cookies are a great favourite with the kids – I can never make enough of them!

4 oz (100 g) sunflower margarine
4 oz (100 g) sugar
4 oz (100 g) plain flour
4 oz (100 g) peanuts, chopped
a little milk

Preheat the oven to 190°C/375°F/gas mark 5. Cream together the margarine and the sugar, sift in the flour and add the peanuts. Mix to a stiff paste with a little milk if necessary. Form into small marble-sized balls, place on a baking sheet, well spaced to allow them to spread. Flatten the tops with the back of a fork. Cook for 15 minutes until browned. Cool on a rack.

Banana and Pineapple Cake

A deliciously gooey cake which is sensational in a picnic hamper. Pack it securely in foil and then in cling-film, so that none of the scrumptious juices escape!

4 oz (100 g) can pineapple
2 oz (50 g) sunflower margarine
2 oz (50 g) brown sugar
2 oz (50 g) nuts, chopped

For the batter
3 oz (75 g) sunflower margarine
5 oz (150 g) sugar
1 egg, beaten
8 oz (225 g) plain flour
2 tsp baking powder
pinch of salt
8 fl oz (250 ml) milk
1 banana, mashed

Preheat the oven to 180°C/350°F/gas mark 4. To make the batter, cream the margarine with the sugar, then add the beaten egg. Sift together the flour, baking powder and pinch of salt, and add to the mixture gradually with the milk, beating all the time. Fold in the mashed banana.

Drain the pineapple and crush it. Melt the margarine and pour it into an 8 inch (20 cm) square baking tin. Sprinkle the brown sugar over it, then add the pineapple and nuts. Pour the batter over the top and bake for 25–30 minutes. Allow to cool, then cut into squares.

BANANA BREAD

For picnic teas, for lunch boxes, or for any other occasion come to that . . . This banana bread is sensationally moist and tasty, and disappears like the melting snow. Use half white and half wholemeal flour if liked.

4 oz (100 g) sunflower margarine
8 oz (225 g) caster sugar
2 eggs, beaten
3 bananas, mashed
8 oz (225 g) plain flour
1 tsp bicarbonate of soda
1 tsp salt
2 oz (50 g) walnuts, chopped

Preheat the oven to 180°C/350°F/gas mark 4. Cream the margarine with the sugar, then gradually beat in the beaten eggs. Add the mashed bananas and mix well. Sift the dry ingredients into a bowl, then fold in the other mixture until well blended. Mix in the nuts and turn into a greased 1 lb (450 g) loaf tin. Bake for 40–45 minutes, until a sharp knife inserted in the centre comes out clean. Cool on a rack before turning out.

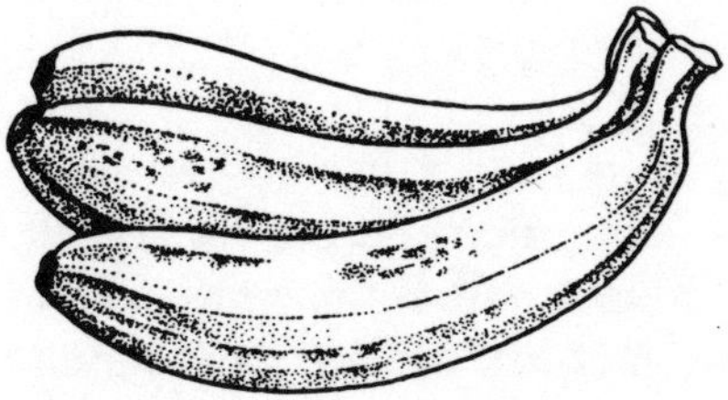

Rosy Apple Yogurt

A brilliant dessert for lunch boxes or picnics, this refreshing variation on fruit yogurt is always popular.

8 oz (225 g) red eating apples
$\frac{1}{4}$ pint (150 ml) thick yogurt
$1\frac{1}{2}$ oz (40 g) icing sugar, sifted
pinch of salt
2 tbs lemon juice

Grate the apples on a medium grater. Mix together the yogurt, sifted sugar and pinch of salt. Mix in the grated apple and lemon juice. Chill, and serve in glasses.

Chocolate Marshmallow Pie

A centrepiece for a picnic with the kids, this wicked pie goes down a treat every time. A fitting finale at a special 'alfresco' meal – but not for everyday (unfortunately!).

Chocolate Biscuit Crust (see page 155)
7 fl oz (200 ml) milk
4 oz (100 g) marshmallows
$\frac{1}{4}$ pint (150 ml) double cream, whipped
2 egg whites, beaten stiffly
grated chocolate

Line an 8 inch (20 cm) flan dish with the chocolate biscuit crust. Warm the milk, then add the marshmallows and stir until they melt. Remove from the heat and leave for about half an hour until half-set, beating from time to time.

Fold in the whipped cream and the stiffly beaten egg whites. Turn into the flan case and leave to set in the refrigerator. Decorate with grated chocolate.

Fireside Teas

Teatime is part of the fabric of childhood: the smell of hot scones fresh from the oven, fresh cookies baked that afternoon, and the home-made chocolate cake which epitomises happiness. Memories of helping cut out gingerbread men, of the first dreadfully messy attempts to roll out pastry, of licking the bowl until it is completely clean of cake-mixture – these remain vivid in later life. What comparison can be made between those home-made teas and shop-bought biscuits and cakes?

Butterscotch Toasties

An old-fashioned treat for cold winter days: banana toast with cinnamon and sugar! Lovely with hot chocolate.

2 oz (50 g) sunflower margarine
3 tbs brown sugar
½ tsp cinnamon
8 slices buttered bread
4 bananas, sliced

Cream together the sunflower margarine, sugar and cinnamon. Spread four slices of buttered bread with the mixture, cover with the sliced banana, then top with a second slice of buttered bread. Grill until toasted on both sides.

Little Miss Muffins

Warm from the oven, these muffins are mouth-wateringly light. The dough is also used in recipes on pages 58, 69, 70, 84 and 114.

Makes 8–10 muffins

6 oz (175 g) plain flour
2 oz (50 g) wholemeal flour
4 tsp baking powder
1 tsp salt
1 oz (25 g) sunflower margarine
6 fl oz (175 ml) milk

Preheat the oven to 230°C/450°F/gas mark 8. Sift the dry ingredients together and lightly rub in the sunflower margarine. Stir in the milk quickly and knead until light. Roll out on a floured board to ¾ inch (2 cm) thick, and cut into circles with a cutter or small glass. Bake for 10–15 minutes until risen and golden brown.

Drop Scones

Kids love these hot, straight from pan to plate. Wonderful food for chilly days in autumn and winter.

Makes 10–12

6 oz (175 g) plain flour
2 oz (50 g) wholemeal flour
½ tsp salt
1 tsp bicarbonate of soda
2 tsp cream of tartar
1 oz (25 g) caster sugar
1 tbs golden syrup
6 fl oz (175 ml) milk
2 eggs

Sift the flours, salt, bicarbonate of soda and cream of tartar into a bowl and add the sugar. Mix and then make a well in the centre. Warm the syrup and milk together, lightly beat the eggs, and pour both into the centre of the dry ingredients. Mix with a wooden spoon until the batter is the consistency of thick cream.

Lightly grease a heavy pan and heat on top of the stove until moderately warm. Drop spoonfuls of batter on to the hot surface. Cook until the bubbles begin to rise, then turn over and brown on the other side. Serve immediately with butter.

Cream Cheese Pancakes

A variation of the drop scone, these creamy pancakes are smooth and satisfying, delicious with the marrow and pineapple jam on page 140.

Makes 12

4 oz (100 g) low-fat cream cheese
2 eggs, separated
2 tbs sugar
½ tsp salt
milk
2 oz (50 g) plain flour, sifted
sunflower margarine

Mash the cream cheese until it is smooth. Add the egg yolks, sugar and salt. Stir in some milk alternately with the flour and mix to a smooth batter. Beat the egg whites stiffly and fold in.

Heat some margarine in a frying pan until it sizzles. Drop in a tablespoon of the batter and cook on both sides until golden. Spread liberally with butter and eat straight from the pan, sprinkled with sugar.

Sweet Toasted Sandwiches

Use fillings such as lemon curd, mashed banana, or jam mixed with chopped nuts, and grill the sandwich on both sides until toasted.

Cinnamon Toast

This is always a popular treat. Simply sprinkle cinnamon and a little caster sugar (or crunchy brown sugar) on to hot buttered toast.

Malt Bread

Moist and gooey, this irresistible bread is a teatime treat, spread lightly with butter or sunflower margarine.

8 oz (225 g) self-raising flour
4 tsp salt
1 oz (25 g) brown sugar
2 oz (50 g) raisins
1 oz (25 g) walnuts, chopped
2 tbs black treacle
¼ pint (150 ml) plus 2 tbs milk
2 tbs malt extract

Preheat the oven to 170°C/325°F/gas mark 3. Sift together the flour and the salt and stir in the sugar, raisins and walnuts. Warm together the treacle, milk and malt extract until well blended and pour into the flour mixture. Mix well with a wooden spoon and pour into a greased 1 lb (450 g) loaf tin. Bake for 40 minutes. Cool, turn out, wrap in plastic wrap and leave for a day or two before eating.

GINGERBREAD

England's triumphant contribution to teatime cuisine! This is a particularly moist, dark and spicy gingerbread, and a firm family favourite.

4 oz (100 g) sunflower margarine
4 oz (100 g) dark brown sugar
2 eggs
6 oz (175 g) plain flour
4 oz (100 g) wholemeal flour
pinch of salt
2 tsp ground ginger
1 tsp mixed spice
½ tsp bicarbonate of soda
10 oz (300 g) black treacle
4–6 tbs milk
2 oz (50 g) raisins
grated rind and juice of 1 orange
2 oz (50 g) preserved ginger, chopped

Preheat the oven to 150°C/300°F/gas mark 2. Cream together the sunflower margarine and sugar and beat in the eggs. Sift together the dry ingredients. Warm the treacle and milk and add to the creamed mixture alternately with the sifted dry ingredients. Beat thoroughly. Stir in the raisins, orange juice and rind, and chopped ginger. The mixture will be very runny. Bake in a greased 2 lb (900 g) loaf tin for 1 hour and 10–15 minutes, until a knife inserted in the centre comes out almost clean. When cold, turn out and wrap in foil or plastic wrap and eat the next day. It stores very well in the refrigerator.

BEST BROWNIES

I've probably made more brownies for my kids over the years than any other recipe. They love them, so do their friends – I've never known a child refuse one!

Makes 12

2 eggs
4 oz (100 g) caster sugar
2½ oz (65 g) sunflower margarine
5 oz (150 g) plain cooking chocolate, grated
1 tbs cocoa powder
2 oz (50 g) plain flour
1 tsp baking powder
3 oz (75 g) raisins or sultanas

Preheat the oven to 180°C/350°F/gas mark 4. Beat the eggs and the sugar until thick and pale. Melt the sunflower margarine with the chocolate and sift together the cocoa, flour and baking powder. Beat all the ingredients together. Add the raisins. Pour into a greased 2 lb (1 kg) loaf tin and bake for 25–30 minutes, until a knife inserted in the centre comes out clean. Cool in the tin on a rack and cut into squares. Remove from the tin when nearly cold.

Infallible Meringues

Foolproof and miraculous: using only one egg white, this recipe makes two baskets or a great pile of individual meringues.

1 egg white
pinch of salt
2 tbs boiling water
8 oz (225 g) caster sugar

Preheat the oven to 150°C/300°F/gas mark 2. Lightly beat the egg white with an electric beater. Add all the other ingredients and beat over a bowl of hot water until fluffy. Off the heat, beat thoroughly for another 2 minutes. Put in spoonfuls on a lightly greased baking sheet, or make two 7 inch (18 cm) circles, and bake for 1 hour.

As a variation, add 2 oz (50 g) chopped and roasted hazelnuts to the mixture.

Biscuit Cake

A really useful recipe which I have used endlessly over the years. If you don't have enough biscuits to hand you can use a little muesli to make up the difference.

4 oz (100 g) sunflower margarine
1 tbs golden syrup
8 oz (225 g) digestive biscuits, crushed
3 oz (75 g) glacé cherries, chopped
2 oz (50 g) chopped nuts and sultanas
3 oz (75 g) plain chocolate, melted

Melt the sunflower margarine with the syrup and add the biscuit crumbs, chopped cherries, nuts and sultanas. Press into a greased cake tin to set and pour melted chocolate over the top when cold.

Nutteroons

Light, nutty biscuits which are crumbly and very moreish.

Makes 12

6 oz (175 g) plain flour
2 oz (50 g) rice flour or semolina
2 oz (50 g) sugar
1 tsp salt
2 oz (50 g) flaked or nibbed almonds
5 oz (150 g) sunflower margarine

Preheat the oven to 180°C/350°F/gas mark 4. Sift the flour s and add the other dry ingredients. Work in the sunflower margarine until a pliable dough is formed, then knead until smooth. Roll out to a thickness of ⅛ inch (3 mm) and cut into rounds. Bake for 10 minutes or until lightly browned.

Sugar Crisps

These turn out lacy, like brandy snaps, and are wonderfully easy to make. Delicious at teatime, and also to go with ice cream after a meal.

Makes 12–15

2 oz (50 g) sunflower margarine
2 oz (50 g) sugar
2 oz (50 g) plain flour
1 tsp vanilla essence
1–2 tsp milk

Preheat the oven to 180°C/350°F/gas mark 4. Cream together the sunflower margarine and the sugar. Sift in the flour, and mix well. Add the vanilla essence and the milk and blend until smooth, then roll little teaspoonfuls of the dough into small balls, and put on a greased baking sheet. Flatten the tops and bake for 10–12 minutes until golden. Cool on a rack.

Oatmeal Cookies

The wholesome texture and flavour of oatmeal makes these cookies lovely teatime food.

Makes 20

4 oz (100 g) wholemeal flour
¼ tsp salt
1 tsp baking powder
4 oz (100 g) sunflower margarine
4 oz (100 g) sugar
2 eggs
1 tsp vanilla essence
6 oz (175 g) medium oatmeal

Preheat the oven to 180°C/350°F/gas mark 4. Sift together the flour, salt and baking powder. Cream together the sunflower margarine and the sugar. Beat the eggs and add alternately with the flour to the creamed sunflower margarine, mixing well. Beat in the vanilla and the oatmeal. Put tablespoons on to a greased baking sheet and flatten the tops with a fork. Bake for 15 minutes.

Ginger Cookies

These ever-popular cookies are a great standby for the biscuit tin.

Makes 20

1 tbs bicarbonate of soda
1 tbs hot water
6 oz (175 g) sunflower margarine
4 oz (100 g) brown sugar
2 eggs
6 oz (175 g) plain flour
4 tbs ground ginger
salt

Preheat the oven to 180°C/350°F/gas mark 4. Dissolve the bicarbonate of soda in the hot water. Cream the fat with the sugar, then beat in the eggs and the soda. Sift together the flour, ginger and salt, and beat into the mixture a little at a time. Drop teaspoonfuls of the mixture 2 inches (5 cm) apart on to a greased baking sheet and bake for 20 minutes.

Smiley Biscuits

The Nutteroons recipe on page 125 lends itself beautifully to making Smiley Biscuits. Roll out the dough and cut it into rounds, then make smiley faces using chopped nuts or currants for the eyes, and cutting a wide grin out of the bottom of the circle.

Maryland Cookies

These chocolate chip cookies make a special teatime treat.

Makes 10

4 oz (100 g) sunflower margarine
1 oz (25 g) caster sugar
2 oz (50 g) brown sugar
1/4 tsp vanilla essence
1 egg
4 oz (100 g) plain flour
1/4 tsp salt
1/2 tsp bicarbonate of soda
2 oz (50 g) chopped nuts
4 oz (100 g) chocolate, chopped into pea-sized pieces

Preheat the oven to 190°C/375°F/gas mark 5. Cream the sunflower margarine with the sugars and vanilla essence until light and fluffy. Add the egg and beat well. Sift together the flour, salt and soda, and add them to the mixture. Stir in the nuts and the chocolate. Drop teaspoonfuls on to a greased baking sheet and cook for 10–15 minutes or until golden.

HEDGEHOG [B]

This party centrepiece is fun to make and a great character who will amuse the kids.

6 oz (175 g) sunflower margarine
6 oz (175 g) icing sugar
2 egg yolks
6 oz (175 g) chocolate, melted
1 box sponge fingers
a little cold milk
grated chocolate
a few toasted almonds and small round sweets

Cream the sunflower margarine with the sugar, then add the egg yolks one at a time, adding the melted chocolate as you go. Mix thoroughly. Dip the sponge fingers quickly into the cold milk to soften them. Make a flat round shape on a plate with the chocolate cream, cover with sponge fingers and continue making these layers until the sponge fingers are used up. Save enough of the chocolate mixture to mould around the outside as you make your hedgehog shape. Cover liberally with grated chocolate. Cut the toasted almonds into strips and stick them in the hedgehog's back. Use little round sweets for its eyes and mouth.

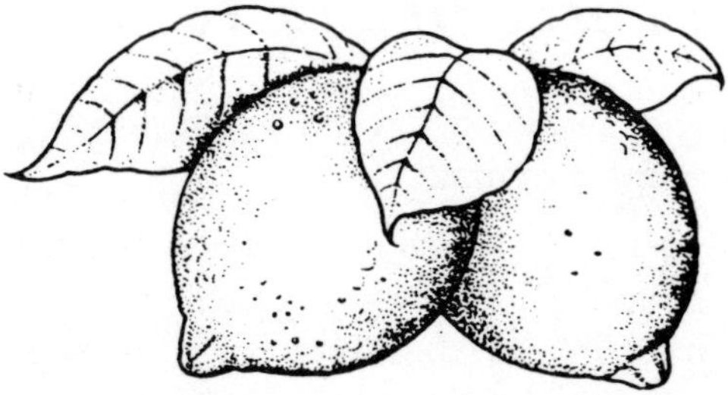

CHOCOLATE CAKE

The lightest and most foolproof chocolate cake I have ever made. We all love it, and it has become almost a member of the family over the years!

4 oz (100 g) plain flour
2 oz (50 g) wholemeal flour
2–3 tbs cocoa powder
2 large tbs black treacle or golden syrup
2 eggs
1 heaped tsp bicarbonate of soda
1 heaped tsp baking powder
5 oz (150 g) granulated sugar
¼ pint (150 ml) milk
¼ pint (150 ml) sunflower oil

Preheat the oven to 170°C/325°F/gas mark 3. Beat all the ingredients together in a bowl. Pour into two greased and floured 8 inch (20 cm) cake tins and bake for 35–45 minutes or until a sharp knife inserted in the centre comes out clean. Turn out of the tins on to a cooling rack and sandwich with jam when cold.

Ice with chocolate spread, or with the wonderful icing that follows, on page 131.

DIANA'S CHOCOLATE ICING

This dark icing has a satiny finish almost like patent leather – and is wonderfully simple to make.

3 tbs golden syrup
3 oz (75 g) sunflower margarine
3 tbs cocoa powder

Melt the syrup with the sunflower margarine, then beat in the cocoa with a fork. Cool a little, beating all the time, and when thick pour over the cake and allow to set.

Yogurt Icing

A healthier alternative to the chocolate icing above!

2 oz (50 g) icing sugar, sifted
1 scant tbs plain yogurt

Mix the sifted icing sugar with the yogurt until thick and smooth. Use as a topping or filling.

Apple Cake

The recipe for this unbeatable apple cake was given to me by a friend in the village, whose house is always filled with the smells of fresh baking. It is delicious – moist yet light, and just as good served hot with thick yogurt as a dessert, as warm at teatime, or cold the next day (if there is any left). It also freezes well.

8 oz (225 g) self-raising flour
4 oz (100 g) wholemeal flour
pinch of salt
8 oz (225 g) sunflower margarine
6 oz (175 g) sugar
4 oz (100 g) sultanas
1 lb (450 g) unpeeled apples, cored and diced
3 eggs

Preheat the oven to 180°C/350°F/gas mark 4. Sift together the flours and salt, adding any bran left in the sieve. Rub in the sunflower margarine. Stir in the sugar, sultanas and apples. Break in the eggs and stir with a spoon. Do not beat. Bake in a large greased cake tin for 1 hour and 15 minutes. Dredge with caster sugar and serve warm from the oven.

Julie's Quick Sponge

Quick and infallible, this easy-to-make sponge is a useful recipe for the busy cook.

4 oz (100 g) caster sugar
4 oz (100 g) self-raising flour
1 tsp bicarbonate of soda
2 eggs

Preheat the oven to 180°C/350°F/gas mark 4. Beat all the ingredients together for 5 minutes. Pour into two greased sandwich tins and bake for about 15 minutes. Sandwich with jam or cream and dust with icing sugar.

Angel Cake

A white, light fatless sponge which is lovely for summer. I often fill it with fresh fruit and simply sprinkle the top with a little icing sugar. It melts in the mouth.

3 oz (75 g) plain flour
2 tsp cream of tartar
6 oz (175 g) caster sugar
6 egg whites
¼ tsp salt
1 tbs lemon juice
1 tsp vanilla essence

Preheat the oven to 190°C/375°F/gas mark 5. Sift the flour. Add half of the cream of tartar and sift again. Sift the sugar and set aside. Beat the egg whites until they form soft peaks. Add the salt and the rest of the cream of tartar to the egg whites. Add the sifted sugar 2 tbs at a time, and then the lemon juice and the vanilla essence. Fold in the flour 2 tbs at a time. Bake in a well-greased and floured tube-pan or large cake tin for 20 minutes, then reduce the oven temperature to 170°C/325°F/gas mark 3 and bake for a further 20 minutes. Remove from the oven, leave to cool in the tin for 10 minutes, then turn out.

Sweet Treats

This is otherwise known as the Sin-Bin, and no childhood is complete without the experience of this kind of sweet sinning. The seven deadlies are all here in their satanic, sugary, sticky guise. Keep them for special occasions and parties, or as an occasional treat.

Yums

Glacé cherries coated in plain chocolate are a dream. For variety, you can add chopped nuts.

Melt some cooking chocolate with a little sunflower margarine over hot water. Coarsely chop some glacé cherries and stir them into the chocolate. Place teaspoonfuls on greaseproof paper to set.

Chocolate Banana Logs

My kids have loved these over the years – bananas dipped in chocolate and rolled in chopped nuts for crunch.

Cut two bananas lengthwise, then into ½ inch (1cm) lengths. Dip in melted chocolate and roll in very finely chopped nuts. Leave to set.

TRUFFLES

This very simple method of making truffles makes a homespun treat which children love.

Makes 12

4 oz (100 g) plain chocolate
1 oz (25 g) sunflower margarine
1½ tbs icing sugar
2 egg yolks
cocoa powder or powdered drinking chocolate

Melt the chocolate in a bowl over boiling water and add the sunflower margarine and sugar. Stir until the sugar has dissolved. Remove from the heat and stir in the egg yolks one at a time. Cool for 12 hours, then shape into balls and roll in the powdered cocoa or chocolate.

CHOCOLATE ORANGE RINGS

Rings of fresh orange coated in plain chocolate are scrumptious, a special treat for after a meal.

oranges
2 oz (50 g) sugar per orange
water
plain chocolate, melted

Peel the oranges and cut into thin slices. Make a syrup by adding a little water to the sugar and boiling it rapidly until it is thick and forms a thread when it trickles off the spoon. Poach the oranges in the syrup, then drain them. When cool, dip them in melted chocolate and put on to greaseproof paper to set. Store between layers of greaseproof paper in an airtight tin.

Marshmallow Roll

This has been a great childhood favourite over the years – and I have loved making it, too!

2 oz (50 g) chocolate
2 oz (50 g) sunflower margarine
2 oz (50 g) icing sugar
4 oz (100 g) marshmallows

Melt the chocolate and the sunflower margarine in a bowl over hot water. Cool a little, then add the icing sugar. Cut the marshmallows into quarters with a wet knife and fold them in. Spread on a sheet of foil and roll it up to set in a sausage shape. Chill. Serve cut in slices.

Toasted Marshmallows

If you are lucky enough to have an open fireplace in the house, this is a treat for chilly winters evenings when the flames are leaping from the log fire. Put each marshmallow on to the end of a toasting fork and cook very briefly in the flames so that the outside is browned and the inside creamy.

Caution: remove from the hot fork before putting in your mouth.

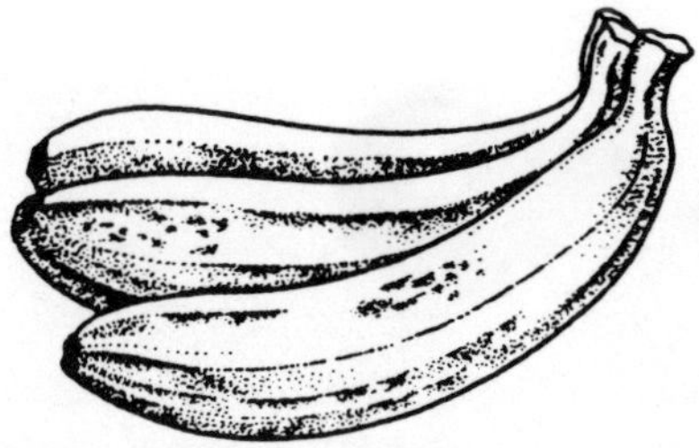

Peanut Brittle

No childhood should be without this!

¼ pint (150 ml) golden syrup
8 oz (225 g) sugar
¼ pint (150 ml) water
8 oz (225 g) dry-roasted peanuts
1 oz (25 g) sunflower margarine
½ tsp lemon juice

Heat the syrup, sugar and water and bring to boiling point. Then cook to 150°C/300°F and add the nuts with the sunflower margarine and the lemon juice. Pour into a greased tin and let it cool. Break into pieces when cold.

Jams and Spreads

No home is truly complete without a shelf laden with home-made preserves. There is nothing like the smell of strawberry jam cooking after an afternoon spent picking them in the sun, or the autumnal smell of simmering blackberries after a walk along the hedgerows. Certainly no shop-bought jam is remotely comparable to your own home-made version.

I have included here just a few of my favourites – the jams and spreads that have proved the most popular with my family and friends, and which are particularly easy to make.

Oranges and Lemons Marmalade

A chunky, fresh-tasting marmalade that is popular with all the family. Perfect on toast, for breakfast.

Makes 10 lb (8 kg)

12 oranges
6 lemons
water
½ tsp bicarbonate of soda
6 lb (3 kg) sugar

Squeeze the juice from the fruit, bring it to the boil with the pips, then strain it. Discard the pulp, then slice all the peel, measure it and put it in a pan with twice its volume in water. Add the juice and the soda. Simmer for 1½ hours until the peel is tender and the quantity well reduced. Add the sugar, stir until dissolved, then boil hard to setting point. Pot and seal.

Sunshine Marmalade

So-called not only because it is full of citrus fruits, but also because – by dint of mincing the peel – it is beautifully easy to make.

Makes 9 lb (4.5 kg)

3 oranges
3 grapefruit
3 lemons
5 pints (3 litres) water
6 lb (3 kg) sugar

Squeeze the juice from the fruit, discard the pulp, then put all the peel through a coarse mincer. There will be about 1 pint (600 ml) of juice, so add this to the peel with the water and the sugar, and cook together for about 1½ hours, stirring frequently, until setting point is reached. Pot and seal.

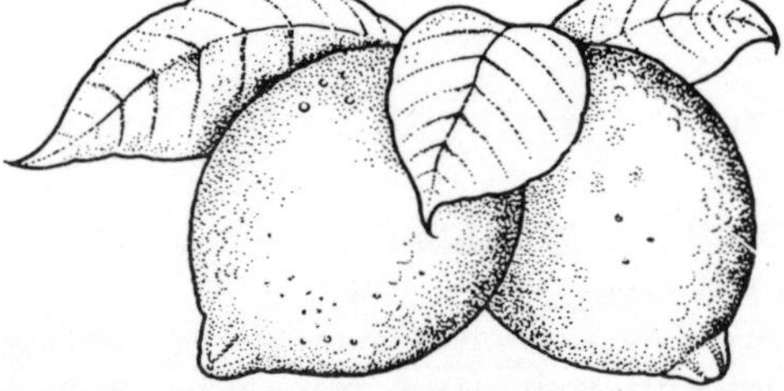

PEAR MARMALADE

A marmalade with a difference, this is fruity and thick, and excellent with early-morning croissants.

Makes 4 lb (2 kg)

2 lb (900 g) ripe pears
2 oranges
1 lemon
1½ lb (750 g) sugar

Wash, core and slice the pears very thinly. Wash the oranges and lemon, remove the ends, then cut them into quarters and slice thinly, removing the pips. Place all the fruit in a pan with the sugar and a little water, and stir thoroughly. Bring to the boil and simmer until setting point is reached. Pot and seal.

PEAR, ORANGE AND WALNUT JAM

This is the best jam in the world. With its wonderful flavours and crunchy texture, it is mouthwatering on fresh bread, muffins or scones, and has a permanent place on my larder shelf.

Makes 5 lb (2.5 kg)

2 oranges, washed but unpeeled
3 lb (1.5 kg) pears, peeled and cored
3 lb (1.5 kg) sugar
1 lb (450 g) sultanas or raisins
½ pint (300 ml) water
6 oz (175 g) walnut halves, halved

Chop the oranges finely. Cut the pears into quarters and slice them thinly. Mix the fruits with the sugar, sultanas and water. Simmer for 1½ hours. Add the walnuts and cook for a further 15 minutes, then pot and seal.

Pineapple Jam

This is easy and convenient to make, and the result is rather exotic. Eat it quickly – it doesn't keep for very long.

Makes 2 lb (1 kg)

1 lb (450 g) can pineapple
12 oz (350 g) sugar

Chop the fruit finely and mix with the sugar and a little of the juice from the can. Dissolve the sugar over a low heat, then bring to the boil and cook to setting point. Pot and seal.

As a variation, make Apricot and Pineapple Jam, using equal quantities of each fruit.

Marrow and Pineapple Jam

This is even more delicious than Pineapple Jam. It has a magical texture and is a marvellous way of using up the annual surplus of marrows.

Makes 10 lb (5 kg)

6 lb (3 kg) marrow, peeled and seeded
1 lb (450 g) can pineapple, drained
6 lb (3 kg) sugar
stem ginger (optional)

Cut the marrow into small cubes, dice the pineapple, and arrange in alternate layers with the sugar. Leave overnight to extract the juice. Add the ginger if you are using it. Boil until setting point is reached, then pot and seal.

Pear and Pineapple Jam

A tempting jam of pears and pineapple is irresistible on freshly baked bread: a teatime treat.

Makes 4 lb (2 kg)

2 lb (1 kg) pears, peeled and cored
1 lb (450 g) can pineapple
1½ lb (750 g) sugar

Slice the pears and dice the pineapple. Add the sugar and a little juice from the can and cook until setting point is reached. Pot and seal.

Angel's Hair

Don't tell the kids, but this is carrot jam. See if they guess: it is sensational.

Makes 2 lb (1 kg)

1 lb (450 g) carrots
1 lemon
1 lb (450 g) sugar
¼ pint (150 ml) water

Peel the carrots and grate them on a coarse grater. Put them with the pared lemon rind, lemon juice, sugar and water into a heavy pan. Boil to setting point, which will be about 100°C/200°F. Pot and seal.

Lemon Curd

I'd had so many failures with lemon curd that I nearly gave up trying, but then I discovered this method and I have never looked back.

Makes 8 oz (225 g)

1 lemon
4 oz (100 g) caster sugar
1 oz (25 g) sunflower margarine
1 egg, well beaten

Put the grated rind and juice of the lemon into a double boiler with the sugar. When dissolved, add the margarine and the egg. Stir continually until thick, then pour into a clean jar and cover. Keeps in a cool place for several weeks.

Peanut Butter

This is so unlike the commercial variety that you would find it hard to guess that they were related.

Melt some margarine and blend it in the food processor with an equal weight of peanuts. The longer you liquidise the smoother it will be. Season to taste with salt and seal in airtight jars.

Delectable Drinks

Home-made drinks are infinitely superior to shop-bought varieties, and you know exactly what goes into them. There are recipes here for juices, cordials and shakes. Kids love shakes and you can improvise endlessly, depending on what's to hand. Use yogurt, buttermilk or skimmed milk as the bases and add ice cream for a special treat. Select the fresh soft fruits of the season, and sweeten to taste, with honey or sugar if needed.

Apple Juice

For windfall time, to make the most of autumn's bountiful harvest.

Simply chop your apples coarsely, removing any rotten parts – any old windfalls will do. Put them into a large pan and cover them with water. Simmer until the fruit is soft and pulpy. Strain through a linen tea-towel or jelly-bag for several hours or overnight. Add sugar to taste and stir until dissolved. Bottle and store in screw-top jars or bottles. Dilute if necessary with soda water. Store in the refrigerator for up to a week.

Orange Juice

Deliciously fresh-tasting, home-made orange juice is incomparable with the commercial variety. Try it and see!

2 oranges
1½ pints (900 ml) water
12 oz (350 g) sugar
1 tsp citric acid

Thinly peel the oranges, leaving the pith behind. Then remove all of the white pith from around the orange. Discard the pith and any pips. Liquidise the pulp and peel, and strain. Discard the contents of the sieve. Boil the water and sugar for 5 minutes. Pour the hot syrup on to the strained liquid, add the citric acid and bottle. It will keep for up to a month in the refrigerator.

Raspberry Cordial

One of summer's best treats, when the raspberry harvest is plentiful. It keeps for 2–3 days in the refrigerator.

Simmer some raspberries with a little water until they are mushy. Liquidise them, then sieve to separate the pips from the pulp. Sweeten the pulp to taste and dilute with sparkling mineral water until it is the correct consistency for drinking.

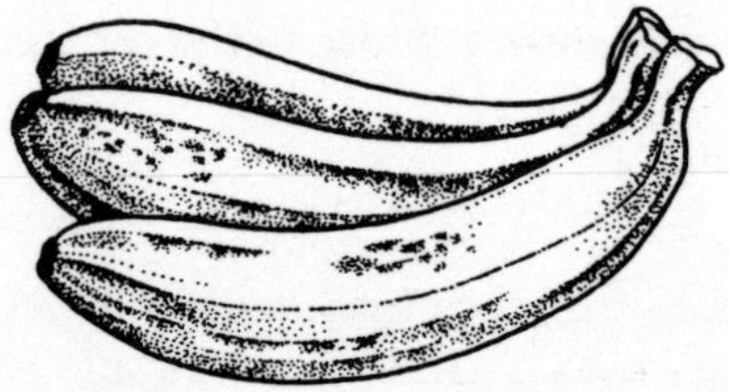

FROTHY MILK SHAKE Ⓒ

Kids invariably love milk shakes, and with home-made ones you can be sure that nothing artificial goes into them.

Per person
1 ripe banana
½ pint (300 ml) skimmed milk
1 tbs ice cream

Cut the bananas up and liquidise with the milk. Put the ice cream in tall glasses and pour the milk shake over.

You can make a Strawberry Milk Shake in much the same way – wash and hull the strawberries before adding them to the milk, and sweeten to taste with icing sugar before pouring over the ice cream.

YOGURT SHAKE

A shake with a difference, the 'healthy' variety perhaps. It is cooling and quenching, ideal for long hot days in summer.

Serves 2

8 oz (225 g) raspberries or blueberries, washed
8 oz (225 g) plain low-fat yogurt
2–3 tbs caster sugar
iced water

Put the prepared fruit into the liquidiser bowl with the yogurt. Blend until very smooth and liquid. Sweeten to taste, and serve chilled, thinned out with iced water.

Buttermilk Strawberry Shake Ⓒ

Buttermilk makes a very light 'shake', and the combination with strawberries is irresistible.

Per person
3 oz (75 g) strawberries, washed and hulled
½ pint (300 ml) buttermilk
icing sugar to taste

Put the strawberries and buttermilk into the liquidiser and blend until smooth. Sweeten to taste, and serve.

Summer Quencher

A wonderfully refreshing summer drink for hot weather, equally popular with kids and with adults. Serve it with ice, in long tumblers.

Makes 2 pints (1.2 litres)

1 pint (600 ml) lemonade
1 pint (600 ml) apple juice
chopped mixed fruit of your choice
a few mint leaves

Chill both the lemonade and the apple juice. Mix them together in a large jug, and float the chopped fruit on top. Garnish with mint leaves and it is ready to serve.

Mixed Fruit Drink

To ring the changes for summer drinks I often mix fruit drinks together, and it always surprises me how delicious and different they taste.

Makes 4 pints (2.4 litres)

1 pint (600 ml) tropical juice
2 pints (1.2 litres) red or white grape juice
1 pint (600 ml) orange juice
chopped mixed fruit of your choice
sparkling mineral water
mint or borage leaves

Chill all the juices thoroughly. Mix together in a large jug and float chopped fruit on top. Add sparkling water to dilute to taste and garnish with mint or borage leaves.

Peach Refresher

Make this drink at any time of year using canned fruit. Peaches are my favourite, but try pears or apricots too.

Makes 2 pints (1.2 litres)

15 oz (400 g) can peaches in fruit juice
½ pint (300 ml) orange juice
sparkling mineral water, chilled

Put the peaches with the fruit juice from the can into the liquidiser, and blend until smooth. Pour into a large jug, add the orange juice and dilute to taste with sparkling mineral water.

Basic Recipes

Bechamel Sauce

Makes ½ pint (300 ml)

1½ oz (40 g) sunflower margarine
2 tbs plain flour
½ pint (300 ml) warm milk
salt and pepper

Melt the margarine in a small, heavy saucepan. Gradually stir in the flour with a wooden spoon, then add the warm milk slowly, stirring all the time until the sauce thickens. Season to taste. Simmer very gently over a low heat for 10 minutes to allow the flour to cook.

For a richer sauce add single or double cream at the end of the cooking.

Cheese Sauce

Add 2 oz (50 g) grated cheese to the finished béchamel sauce recipe above.

Brown Sauce

Follow the béchamel sauce recipe opposite, using stock instead of milk.

Sauce a la Creme

Follow the béchamel recipe opposite, using single cream in place of the milk.

Mushroom Sauce

Lightly cook 4 oz (100 g) sliced mushrooms in a little sunflower margarine. Add to the béchamel sauce recipe opposite with the salt and pepper. Simmer for 10 minutes until the sauce is mushroom-coloured. Serve either as it is, or liquidised to a smooth sauce.

Mild Mustard Sauce

Add about 1 tbs mild French mustard (Dijon is best) to the béchamel recipe above, at the end of the cooking time, and simmer for a few minutes to allow the flavours to permeate the sauce. The quantity of mustard used will depend on personal taste as well as the strength of the mustard.

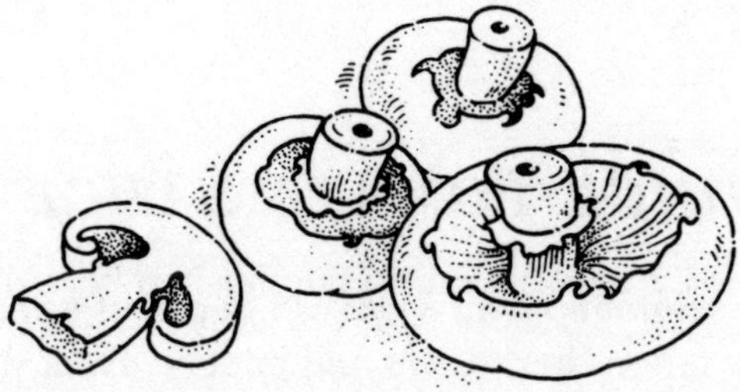

Onion Sauce

¾ pint (450 ml) Béchamel Sauce (see page 148)
8 oz (225 g) onions
melted margarine

Peel the onions and boil them for about 15 minutes until soft. Chop them finely and toss in a little melted margarine. Stir into the béchamel sauce and simmer for 5–8 minutes.

Tomato Sauce

Makes about 1½ pints (900 ml)

1 large onion, chopped
2 carrots, peeled and chopped
2 oz (50 g) sunflower margarine
14 oz (400 g) can tomatoes, chopped
mixed dried herbs
½ pint (300 ml) stock
salt and pepper

Sauté the onion and carrot in the sunflower margarine until they are soft – about 10 minutes. Add the tomatoes and their juices to the pan with the herbs, and cook for a further 5 minutes. Add the stock and simmer for about 10 minutes, until the vegetables are tender. Season to taste and liquidise.

Very Quick Tomato Sauce

Liquidise the contents of an 8 oz (225 g) can of tomatoes with 1 large spring onion, herbs, salt and pepper. Heat through.

VINAIGRETTE

1 tbs wine or tarragon vinegar
1 tsp mild mustard
salt and pepper
crushed garlic (optional)
¼ pint (150 ml) olive oil

Mix the vinegar and mustard in a small bowl and season with salt and pepper. Add crushed garlic to taste, if you want to include it as flavouring. Add the olive oil gradually in a thin stream, stirring all the time until the vinaigrette thickens and amalgamates. Leave to stand for a while before dressing the salad, so that the flavours permeate the oil.

MAYONNAISE

2 egg yolks
1 tsp dry mustard
salt and pepper
½ pint (300 ml) olive oil

Put the egg yolks into the blender and add the mustard, salt and pepper. Liquidise slowly, then with the machine still switched on pour a thin stream of oil into the eggs through the hole in the top of the lid. Stop pouring from time to time to let the mixture thicken. When all the oil is used up and the mayonnaise is thick, pour into a screw-top jar. Keep in the refrigerator for up to a week.

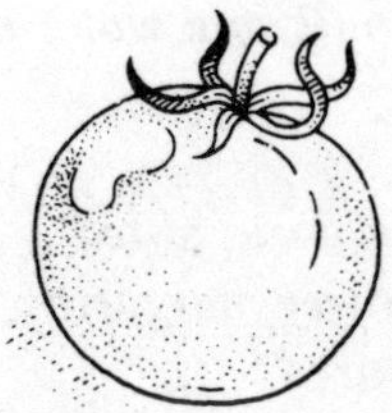

GARLIC BUTTER

One of the classics, garlic butter is lovely on plain steamed vegetables, and of course garlic bread is a treat that never fails to delight the kids. Simply cut a French loaf down the middle and spread liberally with garlic butter. Wrap tightly in foil and bake at 180°C/350°F/gas mark 4 for 15 minutes. Slice and serve.

2 oz (50 g) unsalted butter or sunflower margarine
1 clove garlic, peeled and crushed

Melt the butter or margarine in a pan and add the crushed clove of garlic. Stir for a few minutes, then leave to settle for a while. Chill to set.

BEURRE NOISETTE

For such a simple sauce this has an incredible flavour, and is worth trying with recipes such as the Chicken Kebabs on page 63.

Melt some butter in a pan over a gentle heat and cook until it foams and turns a lovely nut-brown colour. Serve at once.

PANCAKE BATTER

Makes 18–20 pancakes

3/4 pint (450 ml) milk and water mixed
4 eggs
1/2 tsp salt
8 oz (225 g) plain flour, sifted
2 oz (50 g) sunflower margarine, melted
extra milk if required

Liquidise the milk and water, eggs and salt, then add the flour and the melted margarine. Blend for 1 minute. Thin out with more milk if necessary. Cover, and chill for 2 hours before using.

To make dessert pancakes, add a little sugar and use a thin batter.

The pancakes can be made in batches and frozen between pieces of foil.

To Bake Blind

Line the pastry case with a piece of foil, and fill it with dried beans. Bake at 180°C/350°F/gas mark 4 for 20 minutes. Remove the foil and return the pastry to the oven for a few minutes to crisp up.

Oil Pastry

For an 8 inch (20 cm) flan case

6 oz (175 g) plain flour
½ tsp salt
5 tbs sunflower oil
1½ tbs water

Sift the flour and the salt, then stir in the oil and the water. Mix well and knead briefly until smooth. Do not chill or roll out. Press around the greased flan dish with your knuckles and bake blind (see above).

Shortcrust Pastry

For an 8 inch (20 cm) flan case

4 oz (100 g) plain flour
large pinch of salt
2 oz (50 g) hard margarine
3–4 tbs cold water

Sift the flour with the salt, then rub in the margarine lightly until it resembles fine breadcrumbs. Mix in the water and knead to a smooth dough on a cool surface. Cover and chill before using.

Savoury Crumb Crust

For an 8 inch (20 cm) flan case

1½ oz (40 g) sunflower margarine
4 oz (100 g) cheese biscuit crumbs
salt

Melt the margarine and add to the crumbs with the salt. Press into a greased flan dish and chill. Best with a cold filling, but it can also be cooked.

Sweet Pastry Crust

For an 8 inch (20 cm) flan case

3 oz (75 g) hard margarine
6 oz (175 g) plain flour
3 tsp caster sugar
3–4 tbs cold water

Rub the margarine into the flour until it resembles crumbs, then add the sugar and mix well. Add the water and knead the pastry on a floured surface until it is light and smooth. Chill for 2 hours before rolling out.

BISCUIT CRUST

For a 10 inch (25 cm) flan case

8 oz (225 g) digestive or other plain biscuits
4 oz (100 g) sunflower margarine
2–3 tbs sugar

Crush the biscuits to fine crumbs (you can do this in the blender), and melt the margarine. Add the sugar to the crumbs, then mix well with the melted margarine. Press into a greased flan dish and chill.

For variety you can add chopped nuts or grated chocolate to the crumbs before mixing with the margarine.

CHOCOLATE BISCUIT CRUST

For an 8–10 inch (20–25 cm) flan case

12 digestive biscuits
3 oz (75 g) sunflower margarine
2 tbs brown sugar
2 oz (50 g) plain chocolate, grated

Crush the biscuits to fine crumbs. Melt the margarine, sugar and grated chocolate and mix well with the crumbs. Press into a greased flan dish and chill.

Menu and Party Suggestions

Here are some ideas for complete meals, worked out in terms of balance and flavour, to save you having to think! Some are obviously more substantial than others, and this is usually evident from the recipe titles.

On pages 165–6 are ideas for children's parties.

☆ Menu Suggestions ☆

1

Creamy Broccoli Soup
Emergency Loaf

*

Nutty Meat Balls
Lip-Licking Ways with Carrots

*

Apple Cornflake Crumble

2

Corn Cauldron

*

Tuna Noodle Doodle
peas

*

Gooseberry Grunt

3

Midwinter Soup

*

Cock a Doodle Noodles

Lip-Licking Ways with Lettuce

*

Banana Ice Cream

4

Carrot Soup

*

Toad's Surprise

Lip-Licking Ways with Cabbage

*

Banana Frost and Fire

5

Rodeo Spaghetti

Fried Cabbage and Nuts

*

Peach Ice Cream

6

Potato Ring

carrots

*

Topsy Turvy Chocolate Pudding

7

Nice and Cheesy Rice

grilled tomatoes

*

Banana Crumble

8

Onion Super-Soup

*

Toad in the Hall

cauliflower

*

Baked Toffee Apples

9

Crusty Cheese

baked potatoes

*

Banana Fool

10

Mighty Meat Loaf

Tomato Sauce

baked potatoes

*

Paddington's Pie

11

Beautiful Beetroot Soup

Quick Poppy Seed Loaf

*

Zippy Fish

salad

*

Currant Tart

12

Extraordinary Eggs

broccoli

*

Lovely Lemon Pudding

13

Cheesy Potato Bake
salad
*
Banana and Orange Meringue

14

Watercress Cottage Pottage
Bread Fingers
*
Simplicity Chicken
stir-fried beansprouts
*
Banana and Almond Crunch

15

Little Soufflé Flans
peas
*
Roly Poly Pudding

16

Tagliatelle with Vegetables and Crispy Bacon
Brussels sprouts
*
Easy Vanilla Ice Cream
Butterscotch Sauce

17

Tasty Tuna
peas
*
Rosy Apple Yogurt

18

Chicken in the Straw and Hay
carrots
*
Easy Vanilla Ice Cream

19
Spaghetti Rusticana
French beans
*
Yogurt Ice Cream
Chocolate Sauce

20
Cockaleekie
Pasta Twists
salad
*
Knickerbocker Glory

21
Noodle Custards
French beans
*
Pears with Chocolate Sauce

22
Secret Soup
Nutty Pasta with Cauliflower
salad
*
Humpty Dumplings

23
Pasta Bows with Broccoli and Creamy Mushroom Sauce
salad
*
Chocolate Marshmallow Pie

24
Eggs in a Chicken's Nest
cabbage
*
Golden Pear Tart

25
Pasta Bows with Flageolets
salad
*
Peach Crunch

26
Henny Penne
mushrooms
*
Apple and Apricot Crunch

27
Pasta Shells in a Chinese Sauce
salad
*
Flowerpots

28
Spaghetti Carbonara
salad
*
Apricot Charlie

29
Vegetable Lasagne
salad
*
Fruit Stirabout

30
Pink Pasta Omelette
Toadstools
Walnut Bread
*
Easy Vanilla Ice Cream

31

Cauliflower Gratinata
grilled tomatoes
*
Jolly Jelly

32

Igloo Fish
peas and carrots
*
Swiss Roll in the Snow

33

Toads in Cheesy Holes
French beans
*
Ice Cream Cake

34

Roly Poly Pancakes
mixed steamed vegetables
*
Lovely Lemon Pudding

35

Mushroom Fettucine
grilled tomatoes
*
Lovely Layers

36

Leeky Pasta Soufflé
baked potatoes
Funny Bunny Salad
*
Lemon Crumb Pie

37
Lazy Fish Layers
peas, baked potatoes
*
Polar Bear Pud

38
Funtime Fish Flan
salad
*
Topsy Turvy Chocolate Pudding

39
Mole in the Hole
salad
*
Cheerful Cherry Bomb

40
Ham and Potato Bake
salad, grilled tomatoes
*
Gooseberry Grunt

41
Carrot Crater
baked potatoes, salad
*
Easy Vanilla Ice Cream

42
Chuckling Chicken
rice
*
Icebergs

43
Jiving Eggs
noodles
*
Rosy Apple Yogurt

44
Roger's Chicken
grilled tomatoes
*
Peach Ice Cream

45
Pineapple Chicken
steamed mixed vegetables, salad
*
Banana Ice Cream

46
Simplicity Chicken
new potatoes, salad
*
Banana Frost and Fire

47
Sausage Pie
baked potatoes, peas
*
fruit salad

48
Chicken Roll
Tomato Sauce
broccoli
*
Peach Crunch

☆ Party Menus ☆

Here are some ideas for party food. Choose a selection from each category to create a combination of savoury and sweet dishes. Go for as wide a selection as you can – there are bound to be some things that some children won't like.

SPECIAL SANDWICHES

Zebras
Pinwheels
Cock-Eyed Loaf
Pancake Sandwiches

NIBBLES

home-made Potato Crisps
Crisplets
Sunflower Seeds
Peanut Straws
Cheese Butterflies

HOT FINGER FOODS

Crusty Ham
Cheese Dogs
Sausage Snacks
Crisp Tomatoes
Golden Cheese Balls
Fried Cheese
Little Cheese Parcels
Pepper and Bacon Toasties
Crispy Noodles
Barbecue Spare Ribs

CAKES AND COOKIES

Gingerbread
Best Brownies
Little Miss Muffins
Infallible Meringues
Biscuit Cake
Peanut Biscuits
Hedgehog
Chocolate Cake
Angel Cake
Chocolate Marshmallow Pie

Nutteroons
Sugar Crisps
Maryland Cookies

SWEET TREATS

Yums
Truffles
Chocolate Orange Rings
Chocolate Banana Logs
Marshmallow Roll

ICE CREAM SPECIALS

Knickerbocker Glory
Icebergs
Flowerpots
Cheerful Cherry Bomb
Ice Cream Cake
Jolly Jelly and Easy Vanilla Ice Cream

Index